Endorsements

A single, authoritative, highly cited, evidence-based monograph on the COVID-19 vaccines, comprehensive yet concise. Everyone is seeking to understand the mind-blowing reality that government agencies are not protecting Americans nor are they acting in our best interest. This fast-reading text will serve as an invaluable guide ... this topic is bound to resurface in the next few years.

— PETER A. McCULLOUGH, M.D., MPH
Co-author, *The Courage to Face COVID-19:
Preventing Hospitalization and Death
While Battling the Bio-Pharmaceutical Complex*

As a pediatrician who has been on the frontlines of this pandemic from the beginning, I applaud the efforts of Drs. Viglione, Thorp and Sally Saxon in bringing forth the truth about these Covid injections and the corrupt, evil agenda behind them. The fact that the CDC just put them in the childhood vaccination schedule is an unparalleled and unequaled atrocity – a crime against the future of our human race!

— ANGELINA FARELLA, M.D.
*Testified in the Texas Senate hearing to
prevent children from taking part
in an experimental vaccine*

A lot of people will find this book difficult to believe because it reveals evidence that does not comport with their beliefs. Those who are courageous enough to confront the evidence that is hidden in plain sight will be richly rewarded with an entirely new perspective on what might be really going on. It would be hard to read this book and not come to the realization that we've been lied to and that the only way this is going to end is with the call to action articulated at the very end of this book. That's why it's so important that every doctor in America read this book and speak publicly about what they are seeing in their own practices.

— STEVE KIRSCH
Founder, Vaccine Safety Research Foundation

THE COVID-19 VACCINES & BEYOND

Sally Saxon, J.D., and her two medical cohorts, Dr. Deborah Viglione, M.D. and Dr. James Thorp, M.D. have produced a stellar work in exposing, describing and elucidating all the ugly facts that involved the mutiny of medicine for a higher evil purpose. They paint an exquisite big picture of the motives and significance of the greatest propaganda crime the world has ever known. *The COVID-19 Vaccines & Beyond* tells the reader all they need to know to understand why and how we all should oppose the villains of the planned COVID pandemic. Most refreshing is Saxon's acknowledgement of our need to once again become one nation under God as we fight the war against all tyranny. I have nothing but praise and respect for these great truth tellers.

— STEVE LaTULIPPE, M.D.
The first physician to lose a medical license for speaking out against the narrative and successfully treating COVID

The COVID-19 Vaccines & Beyond is a well-referenced MUST READ exposé of the gene therapy agenda and suppression of lifesaving inexpensive safe medicine. Budesonide is the most suppressed secret of the COVID saga. Budesonideworks.com

— RICHARD BARTLETT, M.D.
Discoverer of the successful Budesonide protocol for COVID
30-year GP and Emergency physician
Advanced Trauma Life Support Instructor

Sally Saxon, JD and her co-authors Dr. Deborah Viglione and Dr. James Thorp have created the modern-day Merck Manual for all things COVID, with a particular emphasis on the vaccine. This thoroughly researched, fact-filled book should be incorporated into the curriculum of physician training programs and required reading for all health care providers. Despite the scientific subject matter, the information is presented in a straight-forward, easy-to-read manner, making it appropriate for a wide audience, and I have no doubt it will serve as a resource in the legal arena for actions taken in the wake of the pandemic. I highly recommend this to anyone needing facts to back up their arguments; buy it as a present for your contrarian relatives and propose a debate!

— MARY TALLEY BOWDEN. MD
BreatheMD, Houston, TX

This is a book the entire world needs to read. The lipid nano particle, mRNA technology is a dangerous platform for any "vaccine," and has failed miserably. This book beautifully highlights many of the reasons and data that support this conclusion. It tackles many of the reasons we cannot allow this platform to become the strategy to prevent disease, and why we need to think more critically about what we put into our bodies.

— RICHARD URSO, M.D.
FDA Drug Inventor, Oxervate

As a person who has the expertise to be able to run the largest laboratory and hospital billing operations in the country, I find it astonishing how much the data has been manipulated by the very powerful people entrusted to maintain the Vaccine Adverse Events Reporting System (VAERS). This book is the first to memorialize the nuanced details of this great pharmacovigilance tool, and how it is being manipulated. Saxon, Viglione and Thorp have revealed corrupted tenets, namely, the fact that only *initial* reports of vaccine-injured people are made public, and updated reports to VAERS reflecting their subsequent death are *not*. The knowledge and wisdom contained in this book are a gift to humanity. This read is clear, concise, authentic and shocking!

— ALBERT BENAVIDES
Revenue Cycle Management Expert
Certified Professional Coder
VAERS Analysis Expert

Smart, intelligent and brilliantly put together, a must read for anyone on the front lines of this Scamdemic. The authors have given us a no-holds-barred analysis of what happened and is continuing to occur as opposed to what the government and mainstream media would want us to believe.

— ERIC L. HENSEN, D.O.

As we collectively consider how to navigate both our near and distant futures, living through global medical tyranny and mass deception these last several years, there are two in whom I put 100% trust and faith in: Drs. Deb Viglione, and Jim Thorp. Sally Saxon, JD has held nothing back in this fascinating account and review of the lies perpetrated on humanity that we have come to know as COVID-19. Get ready to learn in this book what to expect as we move forward with our lives!

— DR. BRYAN ARDIS, D.C.

This book is a must read for anyone who is new to the covid vaccine debate or for those who want all the information documented in one place. This book shows this is a war between good and evil, but it does not leave you without hope. It invites you to join the warriors, many of which are in this book. Thank you, Dr. Viglione and Dr. Thorp for being physicians on the frontlines of this war. And thank you, Sally, for working with these two heroes of mine doing the hard work putting this well-researched and referenced book together and for writing about the good news of the "Great Physician."

— JOHN WITCHER, M.D.
Mississippi doctor fired
for putting patients first

Drs. Viglione and Thorp are the real deal. From the beginning, when it was costly and risky to oppose the Narrative, these courageous doctors were asking the tough questions and pointing out all the Emperor's wardrobe malfunctions. Along with lawyer Sally Saxon, their fascinating and informative book gives you a front-row seat to the 'real' pandemic. Buckle up.

— JEFF CHILDERS
Attorney at Law

The COVID-19 VACCINES & *Beyond...*

What the Medical Industrial Complex is NOT Telling Us

SALLY SAXON, J.D.

Deborah Viglione, MD
James A. Thorp, MD

© 2022-2023 by Sally Saxon

All rights reserved. No part of this book may be used or reproduced by any means, graphic, electronic, or mechanical, including photocopying, recording, taping or by any information storage retrieval system without the written permission of the author except in the case of brief quotations embodied in articles or reviews.

Published by: Invitation to Destiny, LLC
ISBN: 978-0-9858180-6-7

Cover Design by Anita Carroll

NOTICE

Removal or Retraction of Sources.

If any of the references or links cited in this book have been removed or retracted since publication, readers may be able to find the article or video through the Wayback Machine at archive.org. Alternatively, the same content might be available at other sites by doing a search on appropriate terms.

Corrections

Corrections of any incorrect data, statements or other information are welcome. Readers may submit any corrections to: info@BreakthroughsForLife.com

DISCLAIMER

The content of this book is offered for educational and informational purposes only, and is not intended to diagnose, prevent, treat or cure any condition or disease or to recommend any medical procedure or treatment that may be referred to in any way. Nothing in this book should be construed as legal advice or medical advice for any purpose. Readers are advised to consult with the health care providers of their choice. The authors and publisher disclaim any liability or responsibility for any harm, financial loss, physical injury, or other adverse impact that may arise from reading this book, including any use or application of any information, opinions, conclusions, research findings, or any statements found in this book. How any reader or user may apply, use, react or respond to any of the content is their sole responsibility.

Dedication

First, we dedicate this book to our Creator and Savior, the giver of life, for whom nothing is impossible. He is able to heal all of our infirmities and diseases, enables us to have peace in the midst of the chaos and storms of life, freedom in the face of oppression, and victory over fear, trauma and every negative emotion. Without His inspiration and direction, this book would not have been written.

Second, to the untold millions of people around the world who have been victims of COVID-19 or the injections, and their families, especially those who were unconscionably forced to make the choice between getting the shots or losing their job. Our hearts break for you, but our greatest hope is that you will find the keys to healing, restoration and freedom from fear that you need for a fresh start in life.

Third, to the untold thousands of brave health care professionals, scientists, attorneys, other experts, whistleblowers and patriots around the world who have risked everything to fight against medical and political tyranny. Many of you are named in this book, but for the even greater numbers who are not, your contributions are no less valuable. We will be eternally grateful to all of you for your sacrifices, dedication and the courage you have demonstrated by taking a stand against the tyranny being imposed in the name of public health. We hope that this book will help to advance the cause you have been fighting for, to alert people of the dangers of the COVID vaccines, and to warn them of the bigger agenda behind the COVID vaccine campaign.

Fourth, to the many health care professionals who believed the people and institutions you should have been able to trust to tell you the truth about "all things COVID." Our hope is that this book awakens you to their true agenda, emboldens you to take a stand for what is right, and empowers you to overcome all of the adverse consequences you have suffered as a result of their betrayal.

Sally Saxon: I would also like to dedicate this to my father, a family physician and general surgeon, who would be in this fight with us if he were still alive. I honor him as one of the early doctors to sound the alarm about the dangers of the government's intrusion into health care several decades ago, when not many shared his concerns or passion about the subject. Thank you, Dad, for your early contribution to the cause, for teaching me the value of freedom, and for that part of your DNA that I obviously inherited that motivated me to join in the fight to preserve it.

Dr. Deborah Viglione: To my mother, June Marken Doster, whose life here on earth ended much too early due to cancer. However, it was her journey through cancer that catapulted me into the world outside of "The Medical Industrial Complex." I quickly realized that conventional medicine did not have the right answers to treat or cure her cancer. This launched me into what has turned into a life-long pursuit for real answers to healing the body and living a healthy life free of disease and the adverse effects of aging. Thank you, mom, I miss you terribly. I also dedicate this to my children and my husband who have "suffered" for the cause as well. My "calling" has kept me from spending the time with them that I would have liked to. However, they have supported me and been my biggest "cheering squad!" I love you all with all my heart!

Dr. James A Thorp: To my beautiful bride Maggie, thank you for being on my team, standing by me, loving me, and supporting my precarious path in attacking the evils of the corrupt medical industrial complex. To my Mother and Father, Ken and Molly Thorp. I love you. God rest your souls and I look forward to being with you again. Thank you for instilling in me a desire to work harder, learn more, better serve the poor and deliver compassionate care as a physician. Thanks, Mom, for being a role model for me as a labor and delivery nurse and instilling in me a love for the Lord. Thank you Ignaz Philip Semmelweis, you are my hero and I look forward to meeting you. Thank you, Ignaz for teaching me how to save lives as a physician, to always avoid group think and to eradicate false narratives responsible for killing and injuring patients. You taught me well Ignaz. Thank you, Ignaz for inspiring me to always be involved with meaningful clinical research to better serve my patients. Fifty years ago when I first read *The Cry and the Covenant* by Morton Thompson I could never have imagined that I would be facing an even worse situation in 2022 than that of Ignaz Philip Semmelweis in the mid-19th Century. What has been done, will be done again. There is nothing new under the sun. (Ecclesiastes 1:9).

Acknowledgements

First and foremost, I would like to express my extreme and heartfelt gratitude for the time, efforts, support and contributions of my two collaborators, Drs. Deborah Viglione and Jim Thorp. This book and the related series in an online medical journal would not have been possible without your expertise, input, feedback, dedication, commitment, and support in so many ways. Your contributions have truly been invaluable and nothing short of amazing. No words can adequately express the depth of my gratitude for the kindness and generosity you have shown me personally and what you have contributed to this project in so many ways. Thank you also for your patience and grace in the process. I am greatly blessed by your passion for freedom and the tremendous courage and commitment to truth you have demonstrated by putting your names on a book covering such controversial topics. If anyone were ever in the trenches fighting a war, you are the kind of people they would definitely want at their side. I am greatly honored to have the privilege of working together with you towards such an important cause. The fact our paths crossed at the time they did and the way they did had to be by divine appointment! I love you both.

Another enormous thank you goes to Dr. Peter McCullough who was incredibly gracious not only to write an endorsement, but also to offer to write the entire back cover! How you made the time to do that in your very full schedule, nobody knows, but all three of us are extraordinarily grateful that you found this book to have value and be worthy of your time, effort and endorsement.

We also want to express a very special thank you to all of the other very busy professionals who took the time to review the book and write an endorsement. Your support also means a great deal, and contributes to our common cause. We pray that the book will prove to be worthy of all who have graciously endorsed it.

Another person who deserves a special medal for her contribution to this book, and for going above and beyond, far more than the "extra mile," is our cover designer, Anita Carroll. Thank you so much for your creativity, patience and persistence in designing a unique cover for this book, and for your extraordinary commitment and contribution to this project.

We would also like to acknowledge all of the many physicians, scientists, attorneys, researchers and other experts who are quoted or cited in the book. Without your invaluable work, this book could not have been written. The information and resources you have made available on this subject matter, in your studies, papers, articles, books, interviews, videos and personal communications have been invaluable in trying to awaken the world to the truth about very serious matters which many still do not want to hear. We commend, honor and thank you all for your courage to speak out at the risk of losing so much for which you have worked so hard and long and paid a very high price.

And last but not at all least, we would like to extend a special thank you to those who gave of their time and expertise to critique certain portions or all of the manuscript. You know who you are, and we are extremely grateful for the time you took to provide your valuable feedback.

ONLINE MEDICAL JOURNAL SERIES

Most of the core content of this book is also published as a 4-Part series in a different format under the same title as this book in
The Gazette of Medical Sciences,
an online open access, peer-reviewed medical journal.

Home Page: https://www.thegms.co

This series is listed under "Public Health" topics:
https://www.thegms.co/department-of-public-health

ACCESS TO HYPERLINKS OF ONLINE REFERENCES

For easy access to hyperlinks for all of the online references cited in this book, use the QR code on the right or the "Endnotes Hyperlinks" button at www.SallySaxon.com.

WANT A SHORT SUMMARY of the KEY POINTS of the BOOK?

FOR A **FREE short summary of this book,** scan the QR code to the right, or use the "Book Summary" button at www.SallySaxon.com

TABLE OF CONTENTS

Preface: How This Book Came to Be Written

PART 1: NOT VACCINES, NOT NECESSARY & NOT JUSTIFIED   1

Ch. 1	Safe and Effective? The Most Divisive & Urgent Issue	3
Ch. 2	A Word of Caution & Encouragement	13
Ch. 3	The COVID Shots are Not True Vaccines	16
Ch. 4	Was a Vaccine Even Necessary?	19
	• An Inappropriate Intervention	19
	• COVID Survival and Infection Fatality Rates	20
	• Availability of Adequate, Safe & Effective Treatments	21
	• The Misleading "95% Effective" Claim	27
	• Case and Death Numbers Were Grossly Inflated	29
Ch. 5	Were the Emergency Use Requirements Met?	35
Ch. 6	Why Many Have Not Heard This Information Before: Reason #1	38

PART 2: DANGERS & GREAT HARM CAUSED BY THE SHOTS   45

Ch. 7	The "Most Dangerous Medicinal Product in History"	47
Ch. 8	VAERS, V-Safe and Regulatory Agency Failures	54
Ch. 9	VAERS: The Under-Reporting Factor & Causality	60
Ch. 10	VAERS Data Comparisons	65
Ch. 11	Early Pfizer Documents: "75-Year Delay" & 1st 3-mo. Report	70
Ch. 12	Adverse Impacts on Pregnancy & Breastfeeding	73
Ch. 13	Devastating Impacts on the Military	80
Ch. 14	Data for Those 65 and Older	89
Ch. 15	Dangers of Giving COVID Shots to Children	92
Ch. 16	Adverse Impacts on Athletes	101
Ch. 17	Dangers of the Spike Protein	103
Ch. 18	Destructive Impact on the Natural Immune System	110
Ch. 19	"Future Framework" for New COVID Vaccine Formulations	116
Ch. 20	Pfizer Documents Show Other Irregularities	120
Ch. 21	Moderna's Improprieties	127
Ch. 22	Problems with the Johnson & Johnson COVID Shots	131
Ch. 23	Other Evidence That Raises Concerns About Safety	135

PART 3: INEFFECTIVENESS & OTHER IMPACTS   141

Ch. 24	General Issues Concerning Effectiveness	143

Ch. 25	Breakthrough Cases	151
Ch. 26	Boosters and Variants	156
Ch. 27	Risk/Benefit Analyses	165
Ch. 28	Clinical Trial Data Reveal a Decline in Health	170
Ch. 29	Natural Immunity is Superior to Vaccine Immunity	175
Ch. 30	Reports from Autopsies, the Funeral Industry, and Life Insurance Companies	177
Ch. 31	Other Impacts: D-dimer Tests, the Story That Backfired & Who Needs to Be Protected From Whom?	186
Ch. 32	Why Many Have Not Heard This Information Before: Reason #2	192

PART 4: THE "BIG PICTURE" & WHAT IS IN THE VACCINES — 207

Ch. 33	Why Many Have Not Heard This Information Before: Reason #3	209
Ch. 34	The "Great Reset" & the Globalists' New World Order	217
Ch. 35	Advancing the Globalist Agenda by Deception	223
Ch. 36	Can the COVID Vaccines Change a Person's DNA?	226
Ch. 37	Technologies Relating to DNA & Genetic Editing	230
Ch. 38	Contents of the Vaccine Vials: General Concerns & Blood Samples	235
Ch. 39	Dangers of Certain Disclosed Ingredients	241
Ch. 40	Undisclosed Substances – General Concerns	244
Ch. 41	Strange Objects and Structures	247
Ch. 42	Graphene: Is it in the COVID Shots?	253
Ch. 43	5G Issues	260
Ch. 44	Reflections on Part 4	263
Ch. 45	This is a War	265
Ch. 46	Conclusion	272
Ch. 47	Call to Action From Two Doctors on the Front Lines	274
	About the Authors	277

Preface

By Sally Saxon

*"The rights of every man are diminished
when the rights of one man are threatened."*
The late President John F. Kennedy

What happens when two medical professionals come together with a retired attorney to address one of the most divisive and urgent issues of our day: **are the COVID-19 vaccines really safe, effective and necessary?** This book is a result of that collaboration.

Even though I am a retired attorney, I believe that this book and the other work I am doing in this season of my life are the most important things I have ever done. They are also by far the most challenging. During my years of law practice, I worked for one of the largest firms in Seattle for several years, and later had a solo practice. I burned out not just once, or even twice, but three times! I did not know what I would do besides being an attorney. All I knew was that I could not go on any longer doing what I was doing. For those of you in the health care community who are burned out from COVID, I can relate. Thankfully, there are keys to recovery and a "new lease on life."

I come from a family of physicians and surgeons, nurses, and nursing home administrators. My father, a family doctor and general surgeon, was actually a pioneer of sorts in fighting against government intrusion into the practice of medicine going back to the 1960's. He even wrote about it, both in booklets and a hardcover book in the late 1970's. I was too young and naïve to appreciate his efforts at the time, but he succeeded in instilling in me an appreciation for freedom and the individual rights and liberties that we have enjoyed in America. I later came to appreciate the importance of our freedoms and legal rights to a much greater degree after living and teaching in a communist country for four years. In recent years, it has become all too clear why my father was so strongly opposed to government intervention in health care and felt that freedom from such intervention was worth fighting for. Sadly, our Constitutionally-guaranteed rights and freedoms have been gradually eroded and destroyed over the years. The era of COVID has brought their destruction to new levels.

The motivation behind this book came from a seemingly unending stream of heart-breaking stories of people who have suffered debilitating and career-ending injuries or even died very shortly after receiving a COVID injection.[i] It was extremely troubling to hear of and see the physical effects of their injuries, as well as to hear that their doctors either refused or were unable to recognize their symptoms and condition as vaccine-related. To make matters worse, their insurance companies refused to cover any or most of their medical bills. Many had to quit their job because they could no longer perform their duties and responsibilities due to their physical limitations. This caused a huge gap in expenses versus income which also adversely affected marriages and families.

Despite all of these adverse reports, the shots were still being promoted as "safe and effective." I had already started to research the subject myself to find out the truth of the matter, regardless of where my search would lead. I had been researching "all things COVID" in connection with an updated version of another book I was writing, which was going to include a couple new chapters about COVID. In early 2022, my research and writing took a detour. It went from enough research for just two chapters in that other book to becoming a separate article focused solely on the shots. My original intent was to appeal to health care professionals in my local area to stop the COVID shots because of the great harm they were doing.

The deeper I dug, the bleaker the situation became. I honestly did not want to believe many of the things I was finding. The more evidence I gathered, the greater the difference I found between the government's narrative and the warnings of those alleged to be "misinformation spreaders," including many doctors, scientists and other experts, each with decades of experience. ***Whose report was to be believed?***

My "article" turned into a "booklet." I then did more research. The initial shorter "booklet" turned into a larger "booklet." I had to do even more research. I had run a couple of earlier versions of it by a few health care professionals. They all made very gratifying comments about it. Some were eager to get copies of it right away for many of their colleagues. But I felt that I needed even more feedback and input from some medical professionals.

PREFACE

It was then that I was introduced to Deborah Viglione, MD, board-certified in Internal Medicine, who then introduced me to James A. Thorp, MD, a board-certified Ob-Gyn and a specialist in Maternal-Fetal Medicine. Both are freedom fighters in the medical community. They read the current version of the "booklet" at that time and offered not only to review it, but to be a part of my effort to get the word out to all who would listen.

Dr. Jim Thorp even recommended that I submit my writing as a series to an online, open access, peer-reviewed medical journal! Obviously, I had never even considered that, since I am not a health care professional. From the beginning my intent had only been to focus on making a difference in my local area. *Besides, would an online medical journal even accept such a manuscript?* Some of what is discussed, particularly in Part 4, is not exactly typical of a medical journal paper, even though the three of us all believed that the health care community needs to be aware of this content because it does directly relate to both their professional and personal lives in profound ways.

I did much more research than I had planned. The two doctors contributed not only sections within their respective specialties, but they also provided input throughout the entire manuscript. With their help, and various drafts going back and forth between us over a few months, we submitted the content of this book as a 4-part series to an online, peer-reviewed medical journal. After the journal had seen only the Abstract and Part 1, I was very surprised at the level of interest they showed in receiving the rest of the series. After we finally finished the remaining three parts, they accepted it all, as is!

I am also writing a "companion" version of this for the general public, both for the vaxxed and unvaxxed, which will include other things that are very important for people on both sides of this "vaccine divide" to know about "all things COVID." It will include issues not included in this book.

If my father were still alive, he would probably be writing a book like this himself and doing all he could to speak out against the medical tyranny that both medical professionals and patients have been subjected to since 2020. He would also be very glad that he would not have to fight the battle alone – as it seemed he had to do in his day – thanks to today's brave doctors like Deborah Viglione, Jim Thorp, the others cited in this book, and many others who have put their professional and personal lives on the line to fight for us all.

---

[i] For example, see testimonies at www.RealNotRare.com.

PART 1

THE COVID-19 "VACCINES" ARE NOT VACCINES, NOT NECESSARY AND NOT JUSTIFIED

"The further society drifts from the truth, the more it will hate those who speak it."

George Orwell

THE COVID-19 VACCINES & BEYOND

ACCESS TO HYPERLINKS *of* ONLINE REFERENCES

For easy access to hyperlinks for all of the online references cited in this book, use the QR code on the left or the "Endnotes Hyperlinks" button at www.SallySaxon.com.

Chapter 1
Safe and Effective?
The Most Divisive & Urgent Issue

*"You may choose to look the other way,
but you can never say again that you did not know."*

William Wilberforce
Leader of the movement to abolish slavery in 19th century England

We should be able to trust our government, the media and the vaccine manufacturers when it comes to matters as important as our health, especially when the stakes are literally life or death. ***How then do we explain why countless thousands of experienced physicians, scientists and other experts worldwide have been willing to risk their reputations, their professional licenses and credentials, and therefore their livelihoods, by daring to claim that the COVID shots are neither safe nor effective, but are actually very dangerous-and should be halted immediately?***

Written by a retired attorney in collaboration with two practicing physicians, this book is particularly helpful for health care professionals and public health officials who have been recommending, promoting or administering the COVID-19 vaccines and for those who are treating vaccine-injured patients (whether their conditions are recognized as vaccine-related or not). It explains the increasingly large numbers of deaths attributed to Sudden Adult Death Syndrome (SADS). It gives valuable information for those who have received these injections as well, and explains the discrepancies between what the government has been telling you and what you are actually seeing in the clinical setting. It is packed with important information even for those in the health care community who have been against the COVID shots.

Have you been asking yourself any of the following questions?

- Why are we still dealing with COVID if the COVID shots were supposed to end the pandemic?

- Why are people who have had all of the COVID shots and boosters still getting COVID?
- Why do we keep getting new variants?
- If it is true that the shots reduce the severity of disease, why are so many vaccinated persons requiring hospitalization and intensive care treatment?
- Why the sudden emergence of Sudden Adult Death Syndrome (SADS)?
- Why should a person who has recovered from COVID get these shots when they already have antibodies and natural immunity which includes memory T-cell response?
- Why would so many physicians risk losing their licenses and board certifications by "spreading" what is alleged to be "misinformation?"

If the COVID vaccines are safe, how do you explain the following:

- **Table 1.** Nearly 168 X the annual average # of pregnancy losses that were published in VAERS [2] following COVID-19 vaccines in 20 months than were published after flu shots in the past 32.5 years. (p value < 0.0001) *(the following are the raw data before any under-reporting factor is applied)*

As of August 9, 2022 by type of pregnancy loss	FLU VACCINE Total pregnancy losses since 1990 (over 32.5 years)	COVID-19 VACCINE Total pregnancy losses in 20 months (1.66 years)
Miscarriages (spontaneous abortions) (in 1st 20 wks)	396	3,723
Fetal deaths (after 20 wks.)	90	458
TOTAL pregnancy losses – both types	**486**	**4,181**
Aver//yr of miscarriages	12	2,242
Ave./yr of fetal deaths	2.77	276
TOTAL average/yr. for both pregnancy loss types	**15**	**2,518**

- **50,239 deaths** within 14 days of COVID-19 vaccinations among Americans age 65 and older as of the summer of 2021 (only several months after the rollout) according to the CMS database (compiled by a whistleblower). [3]

- **17,495% increase in heart disease** in children after COVID vaccinations, up to April 1, 2022, compared with monthly averages of "carditis" cases reported from all other vaccines over 30 years [4]
- **Table 2.** [5] **VAERS data (for U.S. only)** comparing adverse event (AE) reports following COVID-19 shots for **1 yr** with the **COMBINED TOTAL of AEs reported for ALL other vaccines over the previous 30 yrs** (before any *under-reporting* factor is applied)

VAERS DATA as of Dec 31, 2021 (For the U.S. only)	30 yrs 1990-2020 for all other vaccinations COMBINED (U.S. only)	COVID-19 vaccines in 1 year (U.S. only)
Adverse reactions	754,900	715,857
Life threatening events	9,903	11,066
Hospitalizations	38,790	46,755
Deaths	5,241	9,778
Permanent disabilities	12,804	11,413

- **Table 3.** [6] VAERS data comparing the numbers of COVID-19 AEs and deaths reported in *1 year* with *the annual average number of AEs and deaths reported from all other vaccines over the previous 10 years*.

VAERS	Annual ave. of prior 10 yrs for all other vaccines	COVID-19 Vaccines for 1 yr. (as of 12/17/21)	% of increase over the annual ave.
Adverse events reported	39,000	701,126	1,800%
Deaths reported	155	9,476	6,000+%

- **80% of COVID deaths** between mid-February and late May, 2022 in Canada were vaccinated persons, and 70% of those were triple vaccinated.[7]
- **2/3 of the 4,526 children** in Pfizer's clinical trial for 6 months through 4-year-olds did not finish the trial. [8] *Why not?*
- **% of increase among the military in 2021** over the previous 5-yr average (DMED data) (increases for several more conditions are included in Part 2) [9]
    - **2,181% increase** in Hypertension
    - **1,000% increase** in neurological cases (83,000/yr to 863,000/yr)
    - **680% increase** in cases of multiple sclerosis
    - **551% increase** in cases of Guillain Barré
    - **487% increase** in cases of breast cancer
    - **624% increase** in cases of malignant neoplasm of digestive organs

We all know that the official narrative of the entire ***medical industrial complex*** is that the COVID vaccines are "safe and effective" and our main source of hope for overcoming the COVID crisis. That "complex" of players includes government, the major media (including social media), Big Pharma, governing medical boards, major medical publications, international health organizations, and others such as Bill Gates who stand to benefit from a massive vaccine campaign. Yet the worldwide contingent of health care professionals, scientists, attorneys and other experts who believe that these shots have caused incalculable injuries and deaths is very large and growing. They have formed alliances and consortiums of hundreds or even up to tens of thousands of members *each*. They have been accused of spreading "misinformation" for contradicting the official narrative and warning anyone who will listen of the dangers they believe are posed by these shots.

Since all physicians reading this have probably received a letter from their licensing and/or certification boards threatening the loss of their medical license or board certification for spreading "misinformation," ***why do you think thousands of highly experienced physicians would put their reputation and livelihood at risk by sharing what is alleged to be "misinformation?"*** It would stand to reason that they would have to have *solid and compelling data or clinical experience to back it up*. ***What would be their motive to "spread misinformation," given that no one is paying them or offering them rewards or other benefits to do so?***

Collectively, medical professionals world-wide who have been accused of spreading misinformation have been successfully treating hundreds of millions of patients for COVID-19 using proven multi-drug and supplement protocols since the spring of 2020. One would think that their highly effective protocols would have been embraced and welcomed by the government before the vaccines were even rolled out. Instead, as the evidence will show, they were dismissed as dangerous and ineffective, including medicines that have been on the World Health Organization's list of "essential medicines" for decades. ***Why?*** Instead of being lauded for their efforts, doctors who have advocated their use have been highly censored, vilified, and threatened with the loss of their licenses, hospital privileges, important positions and/or credentials. ***Why?***

There are many "why" questions asked throughout this book which should raise concerns about the motives of those who are taking actions against well-meaning and highly competent professionals for reasons that make no sense. The motives of the alleged "misinformation spreaders" should also be considered.

Because of my background as an attorney, I naturally approach this subject from that perspective, just as my two physician collaborators approach the subject from the perspective of their training and experience as medical doctors. From an attorney's perspective, motive affects credibility. The lack of a motive to lie, especially at the risk of losing assets as valuable as one's professional reputation, licenses and livelihood, can speak volumes.

Often a client will present an attorney with a particular situation and ask if the attorney thinks they have a case worth pursuing. Sometimes the client does have a good case, but the cost of pursuing it (financial, emotional, time, the impact on one's reputation, etc.) would not be worth it even if the client won the case. However, there are times when there is something of far greater importance and value at stake than what the client risks losing that motivates them to take the risk– even if it means the loss of their professional credentials, livelihood and finances, reputation, and more. **This is one of those cases.**

The physicians, scientists, attorneys and other experts who have been speaking out against the official narrative are supported by a large contingent of the general public who have refused either to take even one shot or the boosters. No wonder governments have even sought the help of social media to censor what they deem to be "misinformation." What is at stake is not only the alleged misinformation spreaders' own professional livelihoods, but the health and safety of the entire world. Part 4 reveals that there is something even much greater than that at stake, which also motivates many of these brave souls.

In reading this book, you are asked to approach this sharply divisive issue from the perspective of a juror in a trial in which the issues are: ***"are the COVID vaccines safe and effective or not, and were they even necessary?"*** A juror is entrusted with the responsibility to carefully and objectively consider the evidence on both sides of the case. If you were a defendant in a case, would you not want your jury to do that for you? Then it comes down to: ***whose report will you believe?***

The government's "case" has already been made in the court of public opinion through the major media, including social media, as well as in many medical publications. This book presents the evidence underlying the claims that are alleged to be "misinformation." It presents information and data from the government's own databases, regulatory agencies, the manufacturers' own documents, and other sources. Those sources include studies and reports by various experts around the world, whistleblowers, former pharmaceutical company employees, the funeral industry, and life insurance companies.

We were told that vaccines, and only vaccines, could end the COVID-19 pandemic, but they did not. We were told that they were 95% effective in preventing COVID-19, but they have not been. We were told that there would be no vaccine mandates, but there were. We were told that the spike protein from the shots stays around the injection site, but we now know that it spreads diffusely through the body. Pfizer documents that have been released show that the manufacturers and the government knew this, but chose to tell the public otherwise. Doctors were left to discover these and other facts on their own. There are many such representations made to the public that turned out not to be true, and many statements and perceptions that do not match reality or make sense in this whole situation.

The evidence will show that the government's and manufacturers' own data and documents tell a very different story than they have been telling the public (and the health care community) about the safety and effectiveness of the shots. This book goes beyond just numbers. It also reveals evidence behind the scenes, from the manufacturers, the regulatory agencies and other sources, that sheds important light on the whole process by which these COVID shots came about. That evidence has serious implications especially concerning the safety of the shots, as well as the trustworthiness of the entire medical industrial complex.

As of late summer of 2022, it seemed there were shifts going on in the COVID landscape which suggested the COVID vaccine campaign may be winding down, or perhaps just changing its focus or its "stripes." There was a new push to vaccinate children as young as 6-months old, and the CDC was still encouraging adults to get or to stay "up to date" with new formulations of the COVID vaccine targeted for newer variants. Despite the ongoing promotions, fewer and fewer adults have been getting the boosters, and a headline in late September 2022 declared: "mRNA shots for kids are dead."[10]

After three months following the FDA's Emergency Use Authorization of COVID shots for children 6-months to 4 years old, it was reported that of the 1.2 million children who had received the first shot, about 70% had not yet had the second one. That means less than 2 percent were "fully vaccinated," despite extensive media promotion. Only about one out of every 300 eligible children got their first dose during the week ending September 14. ***If that trend continues, why do you think so few parents are having their children get the COVID shots or completing their primary series? Have they been noticing the effects the shots have been having on adults, or on other children injured by the shots? Were they noticing unusual symptoms after their own child's first dose?***

Joe Biden even declared on national TV on September 18, 2022 that "the pandemic is over." Whether other government officials, especially the regulatory agencies, agree with him or not is another matter. Nevertheless, some major media voices have started to report about the dangers of these shots and various kinds of damage they have caused. It is also significant that the CEO of Moderna admitted back in May of 2022 that they had to throw away 30 million doses due to lack of demand because "nobody wants them." [11]

However, even if the COVID vaccine campaign has ended by the time some people may be reading this, the lessons to be learned from these shots and their promotion that are discussed in this book have timeless importance and long-term implications far beyond COVID-19, especially for health care professionals. One reason involves the safety of future medical interventions based on mRNA or other new technologies. A second reason has to do with the corruption in the industry and the relationships between Big Pharma, the regulatory agencies and other players in the medical industrial complex that not only impact safety but also raise the issue of the true driving force behind the promotion of certain medical interventions. A third reason is that health care professionals will have a greater understanding of the problems of their vaccine-injured patients. A fourth reason is that this book will help the medical community respond differently to the next threats of an "emergency" or a "pandemic." Other reasons will become apparent throughout the book.

As many topics, information and data as this book covers concerning the COVID vaccines, there is much more that could have been presented. However, the intent of this book is to present enough evidence to stir people to think critically. It challenges readers to question what we all have and have not been told about the COVID shots and the "whys" behind what has been done and what has happened. The information presented in this book seeks to connect many dots where many readers may not have seen connections before.

This book answers the questions above, including how and why we have been massively betrayed. In addition, Dr. Deborah Viglione says that the most frequent question she is asked when speaking to health care professionals on these issues is: **"Why haven't we been told this before?"** Therefore, that very important issue is also addressed, based on three main reasons.

It is the authors' strong conviction that if everyone had been aware of even some of the information presented in this book, it is highly doubtful that the vast majority of people would have chosen to get the COVID shots, even when mandated by their employers and threatened with the loss of their jobs.

In the era of COVID, the health care community has been put between a rock and a hard place. We are very much aware that many have burned out from COVID. Many have already left the profession, or plan to do so in the near future. Others are afraid of quitting their jobs or speaking out at the risk of losing their jobs because they have to provide for their families.

What has happened to the entire health care system and the medical establishment that runs it is very difficult to accept. However, as increasing numbers of doctors have discovered, there are viable options to being employed by a hospital or other group that is part of the "system."

Whether medical professionals stay in, leave or pursue other options as a health care provider, the most fundamental issues described in this book will still affect them and their families. There is no escaping them because certain issues affect *everyone*, not just the health care community. Therefore, the more we are all aware of them, the better off we will all be.

However, health care professionals are in a unique position to play a pivotal role in bringing this devastating COVID saga to an end. We need to shift our focus to helping restore the lives of those (including those within the health care community) who need physical, emotional and mental healing from the trauma of all things COVID. But it has to start with the truth about COVID and the vaccines. *What is the truth?* You be the jury. *Whose evidence will you believe?*

Four Key Issues

This book provides an overview of four key issues that reveal answers to the above and the following questions:

1) Were the COVID vaccines even necessary?

SAFE AND EFFECTIVE?

2) Are they really safe?
3) Have they been effective?
4) What is the "big picture" that the whole COVID-19 saga fits into that is crucial to understanding what is really going on in the world?

Part 1 presents the evidence that the COVID injections are not true "vaccines" and ultimately why a vaccine was not even necessary. It also questions whether the requirements for an Emergency Use Authorization (EUA) were met, and presents the first of three reasons why many in the health care community have not heard this information before.

Part 2 focuses on evidence related to safety and the degree and nature of the harm resulting from the COVID shots. In addition to government data, it includes the results of various studies and important revelations in documents from the regulatory agencies and the manufacturers, as well as information from whistleblowers and former pharmaceutical company employees.

Part 3 focuses on evidence related to the issue of effectiveness of the COVID shots and certain adverse impacts that affect everyone, vaxxed and unvaxxed. It includes reports from autopsies, the funeral home industry, embalmers and the life insurance industry. It explains the second reason why many have not heard this information before.

Part 4 concludes with a focus on the "big picture" that "all things COVID" fit into, which explains the third main reason why many have not heard this information about the shots before. It also explains why there has been such an unrelenting push for everyone in the world to get vaccinated, and why we are really in a war, but not against a virus. In addition, it addresses some of the most controversial issues, such as whether or not these shots can change DNA, dangers of some of the disclosed ingredients, as well as reports of undisclosed materials in the vaccines. It concludes with a call to action by the two doctors to their fellow medical professionals.

---

[2] Analytics of VAERS data provided by Dr. James A. Thorp, August 2022

[3] https://renz-law.com/special-notice-regarding-evidentiary-findings-related-to-the-official-renz-law-covid-19-investigation/

[4] https://healthimpactnews.com/2022/17500-increase-in-heart-disease-in-children-following-covid-19-vaccines-this-is-not-rare/ (April 2, 2022)

[5] VAERS is the CDC's Vaccine Adverse Event Reporting System database; VAERS Summary for COVID Vaccines through 12/31/ 2021;

https://vaersanalysis.info/2022/01/07/vaers-summary-for-covid-19-vaccines-through-12-31-2021/

[6] Dr. Peter McCullough presentation given at Burleson, Texas, *COVID Symposium: A Legal Perspective*, https://www.bitchute.com/video/ab0LnhD8QdMK/ (Dec. 3, 2021)

[7] https://expose-news.com/2022/06/15/vaccinated-4-in-5-covid-deaths-canada-since-feb/?cmid=cd02f5ae-8cfc-48d8-97d2-a6cc37f11d25 (June 15, 2022)

[8] Dr. Claire Craig, https://rumble.com/v1ah75c-dr.-claire-craig-how-the-fda-twisted-the-data-6-month-to-4-year-olds.html (June 29, 2022)

[9] https://www.ronjohnson.senate.gov/services/files/FB6DDD42-4755-4FDC-BEE9-50E402911E02, Letter dated Feb.1, 2022 to Secretary Lloyd Austin, Dept. of the Defense.

[10] Alex Berenson, https://alexberenson.substack.com/p/mrna-covid-shots-for-kids-are-dead (Sept. 22, 2022)

[11] Katabella Roberts, https://www.theepochtimes.com/moderna-throwing-30-million-doses-in-the-garbage-over-dwindling-vaccine-demand-ceo_4489393.html (May 25, updated May 26, 2022)

Chapter 2
A Word of Caution and Encouragement to Those Who Have Received, Given or Recommended the Shots

It is difficult to dive into the rest of this book without us first sharing a few words of both caution and encouragement for those who either have received the COVID vaccines themselves, have loved ones who have, or have been recommending or administering them to others. **Some of the information in this book might be quite disturbing and difficult to accept for those who have trusted the government, Big Pharma, the major media, and others in the medical industrial complex to tell them the truth about matters that literally involve life or death.** It is very difficult to discover, as well as to be the one to tell others, that we have all been deceived and betrayed on such important matters. The truth about these issues may be a "difficult pill to swallow." But especially in the times we are living in right now, the consequences of being unaware or deceived are even more challenging.

Many readers may experience a wide range of negative emotions while reading certain portions of this book as they discover how they have been lied to by people they trusted on matters of such great importance. However, any emotional and mental impacts caused by discovering the truth, as well as from the trauma suffered because of the physical injuries following the shots, can be healed and overcome as well. Truth is the key to complete recovery and restoration because truth, rightly applied, sets people free – from fear, trauma, despair, anger, guilt, regrets and all other negative emotions. We encourage you to let truth lead you to solutions, healing, peace and freedom, and to turn negative emotions into positive action. Without truth or knowledge of the facts, there are either no solutions at all, or only much less than the best. But with them, you can have a fresh start in life, rather than allow negative emotions to dominate, hurt or overcome you.

There are existing protocols that have been shown to relieve at least some of the physical symptoms and problems resulting from the shots. However, every person is different, both in terms of the kinds of damage they have suffered and in their response to various remedies or solutions. In general, these protocols are designed to reduce inflammation, reduce risk of blood clotting, improve and restore the immune system, and help the body heal. The body has mechanisms and pathways to heal from various kinds of organ, tissue, and DNA damage. Therefore, these protocols involve lifestyle modification, dietary recommendations, targeted nutritional supplements, medications prescribed by your treating physician, stress reduction, and spiritual healing and renewal. Be encouraged that researchers and physicians are working diligently to discover more and better remedies.

The resources at www.TruthForHealth.org include a vaccine injury treatment guide listing various tests that may help to diagnose the nature and degree of post-vax injuries.[12] The President and CEO of that organization is Dr. Elizabeth Lee Vliet, MD, who has been a leader in patient-centered care for many years. She has been part of a team of frontline physicians advocating early treatment COVID protocols since February 2020. Other information is provided by the World Council for Health[13] and the Front Line COVID-19 Critical Care Alliance (FLCCC).[14] There are several other sources as well. These resources are continually evolving, as experts learn more about what is in the shots and their effects. **However, some of the most effective treatments may be outside the scope of allopathic medicine. Therefore, patients and allopathic health care professionals may need to look for solutions and help in other areas of health care.**

A very important element of the truth is this: to the extent that the health care community's best efforts and solutions are not able to fully restore physical health and vitality to those injured by the COVID shots, or to help people overcome the negative emotional impacts, **we believe without any doubt that real hope for complete restoration is available to all through our Creator, God, the "Great Physician."** Absolutely nothing is impossible for Him. God is still doing many miracles today, and we believe that our spiritual lives and faith play an essential and important role in healing and restoration, *no matter how impossible a person's*

A WORD OF CAUTION AND ENCOURAGEMENT

situation may appear in the natural. God has even supernaturally replaced surgically implanted steel plates and pins, has created brand new organs and body parts, and totally healed many diseases that doctors have deemed to be terminal. ***Nothing is impossible for Him.***

This is true not only for the physical impacts of the shots, but also for the emotional and mental impacts. For many people, these impacts may be equally challenging as physical injuries, whether caused by the shots themselves or even from learning the truth about them, or both. Fear is destructive to the immune system, it cripples mental health and can lead to emotional paralysis and failure to react or respond in positive ways. Fear also robs us of peace, joy and hope. The major media's lies about the true degree of danger of COVID and the lack of any treatments created an atmosphere of fear and despair designed to lead people to accept their official narrative surrounding "all things COVID," their oppressive counter-measures, and COVID vaccines as their only solution.

Evidence-based faith (as opposed to "wishful thinking") is the antidote to fear. Therefore, we hope you are encouraged by our belief that every kind of negative impact you or others have suffered as a result of COVID or the shots *can be* overcome, whether through health care professionals or by the "Great Physician" directly.

If you struggle with the impacts from what our government, the manufacturers and the major media have lied about and what they did not tell us, what do you have to lose by giving God a chance to prove Himself to you in your time of need? **By the time you finish this book, you will understand why we believe that God's intervention at this time in history is not simply an option, but is actually necessary** – and not only to stop the COVID crisis and to bring healing and restoration to people's lives from its devastating effects.

---

[12] https://www.truthforhealth.org/2022/04/vaccine-injury-treatment-guide-your-roadmap-to-recovery/

[13] https://worldcouncilforhealth.org/resources/a-practical-approach-to-keeping-healthy-after-your-covid-19-jab/

[14] https://covid19criticalcare.com/covid-19-protocols/i-recover-post-vaccine-treatment/

Chapter 3
The COVID Shots are Not True Vaccines

First, it is important to recognize that none of the COVID-19 shots meet the legal or commonly understood definitions of a vaccine. By statute, the National Vaccine Program enacted by Congress in 1986 reveals that the purpose of a vaccine is "to achieve optimal prevention of human infectious diseases..."[15] In another statutory context, "The term 'vaccine' means any substance designed to be administered ... for the prevention of 1 or more diseases." [16]

Prevention is what the public has been told that a vaccine is supposed to do and what the public was told the COVID shots would do. However, the data show that the COVID shots neither prevent the disease nor transmission of it. The data revealing large percentages of "breakthrough" cases of vaccinated persons are presented in Part 3. In September 2021, the CDC changed its definition of a vaccine. It had been "A product that stimulates a person's immune system to produce immunity to a specific disease, protecting the person from that disease." It became a *"preparation that is used to stimulate the body's immune response against diseases."* [17]

When it became clear that these injections were not preventing disease or transmission, the official narrative became that they would lessen the severity of symptoms, and reduce hospitalizations and deaths. This would classify the injections as a treatment, not a vaccine.[18] This claim is problematic for several reasons. The first is that these shots were given Emergency Use Authorization as a vaccine, not as a treatment, and therefore made the manufacturers immune from liability under federal law.[19] To classify these injections as a treatment would remove their liability protection. Key data are also mounting that contradict this claim of reducing severity. Data worldwide reveal that vaccinated persons have accounted for most COVID hospitalizations and deaths for quite a while, especially among the triple-vaxxed.[20] (See Part 3.)

Should these have been more appropriately classified as "gene therapy"? The Complaint in a lawsuit filed by Dr. Devan Griner, MD against Joseph R.

Biden, Jr., the DHHS, and others reveals various reasons why they should. A 2020 filing by Moderna with the Securities and Exchange Commission (SEC), states: "mRNA is considered a **gene therapy product** by the FDA."[21] A similar statement is found in the 2020 SEC filing by Pfizer's partner BioNTech.[22] The FDA's definition of gene therapy products includes "nucleic acids (e.g., plasmids, in vitro transcribed ribonucleic acid (RNA), genetically modified microorganisms (e.g., viruses, bacteria, fungi)…" [23] For more information as to why the COVID injections are not vaccines, see the Complaint in the Griner lawsuit.[24]

The Global COVID Summit coalition, which represents over 17,000 physicians and medical scientists, also considers these shots "genetic therapy injections."[25] Dr. Michael Yeadon, a former Pfizer vice president and scientist, also calls them "gene-based products," saying "they cunningly managed to disguise them under the word vaccine … The only thing they bear in common with traditional vaccines is the word… There's no other similarity." By calling them that, "they were allowed to proceed down a development pathway that's relatively light in terms of obligations on the innovators … *it should have been classed as … genetic medicine where the obligations … are extremely onerous.*" [26]

In a speech at the World Health Summit in October 2021, Stefan Oelrich, head of Bayer's Pharmaceuticals Division, also confirmed that mRNA vaccines are a form of gene therapy. He said:

> "'We are really taking that leap [to drive innovation] … in cell and gene therapies … ultimately the mRNA vaccines are an example for that cell and gene therapy... if we had surveyed two years ago in the public – 'would you be willing to take a gene or cell therapy and inject it into your body?' – we probably would have had a 95% refusal rate.'" [27]

The above statements reveal at least three reasons why it was advantageous to the manufacturers to have these shots treated as vaccines instead of as "gene therapy" products according to the FDA definitions: 1) the liability protection; 2) the less onerous regulatory requirements; and 3) greater public acceptance. In light of the above, subsequent references to the COVID shots as "vaccines" should not be construed as an acknowledgement that they are true "vaccines." (More about gene therapy in Part 4.)

[15] 42 U.S. Code §300aa-1 (1986); see https://www.law.cornell.edu/uscode/text/42/300aa-1 (accessed April 30, 2022)

[16] 26 U.S. Code §4132 – Definitions and special rules; see https://www.law.cornell.edu/uscode/text/26/4132#a_2 (click on the hyperlinked word "vaccine") (accessed April 30, 2022)

[17] *Immunization: The Basics*, https://www.cdc.gov/vaccines/vac-gen/imz-basics.htm (last visited April 29, 2022). (Check the "Wayback Machine" for that website at www.archive.org comparing Sept. 1, 2021 and Sept. 2, 2021)

[18] See Devan Griner, MD vs. Joseph R. Biden, Jr., et al, Case No: 2:22-cv-00149-DAK, Complaint for Violation of Civil Rights and Declaratory and Injunctive Relief, filed March 4, 2022 in the U.S. District Court for the District of Utah, https://static1.squarespace.com/static/61e10985eb59005edbd1b451/t/6222b6d4b8cc1431b30705a0/1646442197434/2022.03.04+Complaint+As+Filed.pdf, p. 16

[19] By virtue of the HHS Secretary's Declaration of Emergency invoking the relevant provisions of the PREP Act, 42 U.S.C. § 247d-6d and 42 U.S.C. § 247d-6e; see also https://www.bclplaw.com/en-US/insights/immunity-from-liability-under-the-us-prep-act-for-medical-countermeasures-during-the-sars-cov-2covid-19-pandemic.html (May 22, 2020)

[20] E.g., UK data: https://dailyexpose.uk/2022/04/12/distracted-boris-kyiv-fully-vaccinated-92-percent-covid-deaths/ (April 12, 2022); Canada: https://expose-news.com/2022/06/22/trudeau-panics-9-in-10-covid-deaths-fully-vaccinated/(June 22, 2022)

[21] *Moderna SE Form 10-q,* UNITED STATES SECURITIES AND EXCHANGE COMMISSION (2020), https://www.sec.gov/Archives/edgar/data/1682852/000168285220000017/mrna-20200630.htm at page 70

[22] *BioNTech SE Form 20-F,* UNITED STATES SECURITIES AND EXCHANGE COMMISSION (2020), https://www.sec.gov/Archives/edgar/data/1776985/000156459021016723/bntx-20f_20201231.htm at page 26

[23] FDA, Long Term Follow-Up After Administration of Human Gene Therapy Products: Guidance for Industry. (Jan. 2020); https://www.fda.gov/media/113768/download

[24] See Devan Griner, MD vs. Joseph R. Biden, Jr., et al, Case No: 2:22-cv-00149-DAK, Complaint for Violation of Civil Rights and Declaratory and Injunctive Relief, filed March 4, 2022 (cited above), pp. 13-22.

[25] https://globalcovidsummit.org/news/declaration-iv-restore-scientific-integrity (May 11, 2022)

[26] Dr. Michael Yeadon presentation, https://odysee.com/@Quasar:3/Mike-Yeadon-Testimony-for-the-Grand-Jury:9 (testimony date Feb. 4, 2022)

[27] Jack Bingham, https://www.lifesitenews.com/news/bayer-executive-mrna-shots-are-gene-therapy-marketed-as-vaccines-to-gain-public-trust/ (Nov. 10, 2021)

Chapter 4
Was a Vaccine Even Necessary?

An Inappropriate Intervention

Dr. Toby Rogers, Ph.D., a political economist whose focus is Big Pharma and regulatory corruption, explains why a vaccine was not an appropriate response to the COVID crisis:

> "Viruses that evolve rapidly are bad candidates for a vaccine. There is no vaccine for the common cold nor HIV because these viruses evolve too quickly for a vaccine to be effective. The SARS-CoV-2 virus is a bad candidate for a vaccine, as it has rapidly mutated, which is why all previous attempts to develop a vaccine against coronaviruses have failed (they never made it out of animal trials because the animals died during challenge trials or were injured by the vaccine)."[28]

Dr. Michael Yeadon, the former Pfizer vice president and scientist cited above who spent 32 years in the biopharmaceutical industry, agrees: "It's never appropriate to seek to invent, develop, manufacture, and distribute a novel vaccine for a respiratory pathogen of such modest lethality, even if it was a bit worse than it is." The reason, he said, is that by the time all the necessary work was done to establish its safety for billions of people, the pandemic for which it was created would probably have already ended.[29]

If a vaccine was not an appropriate intervention or not necessary to begin with, either to end or control the COVID "crisis," this raises a very important question: ***Why then has the medical industrial complex been so hell-bent on getting the entire world injected with these shots?*** The reasons would likely have nothing to do with public health. By the end of this book, you will know the answer. That alone should raise additional issues about their safety and efficacy.

FOUR KEY REASONS WHY A VACCINE WAS NOT NECESSARY

The lack of a need for a COVID vaccine in the first place is supported by at least four key issues (besides the superiority of natural immunity, discussed later):
  1) The very high survival rate of people who get COVID;
  2) The availability of adequate, safe and effective treatments;
  3) The extremely misleading claim of "95% effectiveness;" and
  4) The highly inflated COVID death and case data.

COVID-19 Survival Rates Have Been Over 99.4% for Most People

An article dated May 25, 2020, a few months into the COVID crisis, reported the CDC's realistic estimate of the COVID-19 death rate: "under its most likely scenario, the number is 0.26%." That was almost the same as what a Stanford study had concluded a month earlier,[30] which was 0.12 - 0.2%.[31] In an even earlier editorial in the *NEJM* dated February 28, 2020, on which Anthony Fauci was the lead author, he stated that "the overall clinical consequences of Covid-19 may ultimately be more akin to those of a severe seasonal influenza (which has a case fatality rate of approximately 0.1%) …"[32] Given that many who died were elderly with multiple comorbidities and/or died in nursing homes, that means the infection fatality rate (IFR) for everyone else was even less. Table 4 below sets forth the CDC's data as of the early fall of 2020.[33]

Table 4. CDC's Infection Fatality Rates (and Corresponding Survival Rates extrapolated from IFR), as of September 10, 2020.

Age group	Infection Fatality Rate (IFR)	Survival Rate
0-19 yrs	0.00003 (0.003%)	99.997 %
20-49 yrs	0.0002 (0.02%)	99.980 %
50-69 yrs	0.005 (0.5%)	99.500 %
70+ yrs.	0.054 (5.4%)	94.600 %

A study months later in 2021 by Stanford Professor Dr. John Ioannidis revealed similar results, as shown in Table 5 below.[34] In addition to the rates shown for those under 70, the survival rate for those over 70, the group with the highest rate of co-morbidities, was 94.6%.[35] ***Did the major media tell us any of these survival rates to try to dispel people's fears? Why not?***

WAS A VACCINE EVEN NECESSARY?

Table 5. COVID Survival rates and IFR by Dr. John Ioannidis (July 2021)

Age	Median IFR	Survival rate estimate	Mortality rate estimate
0-19	0.0027%	99.9973%	0.0027%
20-29	0.0140%	99.9860%	0.0140%
30-39	0.0310%	99.9690%	0.0310%
40-49	0.0820%	99.9880%	0.0120%
50-59	0.2700%	99.7300%	0.2700%
60-69	0.5900%	99.4100%	0.5900%

Age stratified infection fatality rates for COVID-19 Ioannides and Axfors July 2021

Dr. Peter R. Breggin, MD, raises another factor that would further reduce the death rate: *CDC's death rates were based on patients who did not get adequate treatment at home, due to government policies.* But for patients who did, "there were very few deaths, even within the older population." Breggin states:

> "...with a very high degree of statistical probability, if you receive proper early treatment, you will reduce your chance of hospitalization by 87.6% and your risk of death by 74.9%."[36]

He also says, as have many other doctors, that COVID was less serious for most than seasonal flu.[37]

The Availability of Adequate, Safe and Effective Treatments

The issue of the availability of adequate, effective treatments is relevant for various reasons. One is obviously how many COVID hospitalizations and deaths could have been avoided by such available treatments. Another important reason is that the very large and growing number of vaccine-related deaths and injuries could have been prevented because the shots would not have been necessary. A third key that will be explained further below is that by law, the Emergency Use Authorizations (EUA) for the vaccines could never have been granted by the FDA if there had been "adequate" alternative treatments available that were ***approved***.

As you surely know, Ivermectin, Hydroxychloroquine and other medicines have been demonized by the CDC, FDA and the major media and were declared to be ineffective and even dangerous in the treatment of COVID-19. However, these and others such as Budesonide, and other drug and supplement combinations have been proven by countless thousands of doctors to be very effective treatments for COVID-19, especially when used in early treatment, or some even prophylactically.

Hydroxychloroquine (HCQ)

One of the first doctors to be successful in early treatment using HCQ to treat COVID-19, in combination with zinc and azithromycin, was Dr. Vladimir "Zev" Zelenko. He had advised President Trump, as well the President of Brazil and other high-profile people in the use of HCQ for treating COVID-19. In July 2020, Dr. Harvey Risch, a distinguished epidemiologist at the Yale School of Public Health, stated unequivocally with regard to HCQ:

> "'The key to defeating COVID-19 already exists. We need to start using it…. When this inexpensive oral medication is given very early in the course of illness…it has shown to be highly effective, especially when given in combination with the antibiotics azithromycin or doxycycline and the nutritional supplement zinc.'"[38]

In fact, the same article in which Risch was quoted further reveals: "The NIH has known since 2005 that HCQ is effective against the Covid family of viruses." It also noted that HCQ has been "in constant use since 1944. It has virtually no detectable side effects." Dr. Risch urged that "'HCQ and its companion medications 'should be immediately adopted as the new standard of care in high-risk patients.'" In 2020, several countries were reporting successful outcomes using HCQ to treat COVID-19.[39] **Why not the U.S.?**

Early outpatient treatment for COVID-19 was discussed at a Senate subcommittee hearing on November 19, 2020 chaired by Senator Ron Johnson.[40] Drs. Risch and Peter McCullough, each an author of hundreds of peer-reviewed papers, were among nine physician-scientists testifying to the effectiveness of early treatment multi-drug protocols using drugs like HCQ and Ivermectin to prevent most hospitalizations and deaths.

Dr. Ashish Jha, then a professor of Global Health at Harvard, argued for the official narrative. However, he did not cite any study showing that early treatment protocols *did not* work. Also, Jha has done no peer-reviewed studies, and unlike the other panelists, who collectively had successfully treated thousands of patients, had not treated any COVID patients himself.

WAS A VACCINE EVEN NECESSARY?

Dr. Stella Immanuel, MD was one of the America's Frontline Doctors group who spoke in Washington, D.C. in July 2020 who tried to assure the public that effective treatments for COVID were available. At that time, she had successfully treated 350 patients with hydroxychloroquine, zinc and azithromycin, including patients as old as 87 and 92. They all got well. In her book, *Let America Live*, she also questions the credibility of specialists who were not even treating COVID patients, yet were making uninformed and false claims about hydroxychloroquine in the media.[41]

Budesonide

Another medicine that has proven highly effective against COVID-19 is Budesonide. Dr. Richard Bartlett is an emergency room doctor in Texas.[42] He also teaches advanced trauma life support to ER physicians. He has successfully treated numerous asthma patients with Budesonide. When COVID patients first started coming into the ER, he gave them Budesonide and their condition improved. He was shocked at how well it worked. Especially because these were patients whom others had written off as "goners," yet they recovered quickly using Budesonide. That was true even for patients with serious comorbidities and risk factors who ultimately did not have to be hospitalized. He added that it is so safe that it has been used on 2-pound babies in the ICU.

Oxford University, which boasts of having 72 Nobel Prize laureates, did two randomized controlled trials which concluded *that 90% of hospitalizations, ER visits and urgent care visits could be prevented with one medicine used early against COVID: Budesonide.* Yet Dr. Anthony Fauci has said that Budesonide "was just a placebo." Dr. Bartlett has seen patients both in early and late stages recover successfully using Budesonide, even in extreme cases. He also cited studies from 2017 on patients on ventilators which showed the effectiveness of Budesonide in improving several symptoms.[43]

Ivermectin

Ivermectin is a Nobel Prize winning drug. It has been used by countless doctors worldwide against COVID-19 with excellent success. One advantage of Ivermectin is that it has also proven to be very effective in all stages of COVID-19.[44] One study that was funded by the WHO with 1,255 participants showed that Ivermectin reduced COVID-19 deaths by 75%. Other studies showed reductions in deaths ranging from 64% to 91%.[45] A summary of the clinical trial evidence for Ivermectin is available at the Frontline COVID-19 Critical Care Alliance website.[46] Also, the most comprehensive compilation and review of Ivermectin studies in the world is found at www.IVMmeta.com. It has real-time meta-analysis of 89 studies of Ivermectin for COVID-19 (as of July 26, 2022), from 960 scientists involving 133,038 patients in 27 different countries.

Dr. Pierre Kory, a lung and ICU specialist, board-certified in Critical Medicine, Pulmonary Diseases and Internal Medicine, is one of the most well-known of the doctors who have had tremendous success with Ivermectin in treating COVID-19.[47] He also has extensively researched the studies around the world involving the effectiveness of Ivermectin. He has used it prophylactically as well as in treating COVID patients at various stages. He is also one of the doctors who gave testimony before a Congressional committee on the safety and excellent results using Ivermectin to treat COVID-19. Noting that he does not use the word "miracle" lightly, he said:

> "mountains of data that have emerged from ... many centers and countries around the world *showing the miraculous effectiveness of Ivermectin. It basically obliterates transmission of this virus. If you take it you will not get sick.* ... The amount of evidence to show that Ivermectin is life-saving and protective is so immense and the drug is so safe, my colleagues have talked about it. . . It is critical for its use in this disease...."[48]

In a different hearing he also stated:

> "Taken together ... dozens of clinical trials that have now emerged from around the world are substantial enough to reliably assess clinical efficacy ... data from 18 randomized controlled trials that included over 2,100 patients ... demonstrated that Ivermectin produces faster viral clearance, faster time to hospital discharge, faster time to clinical recovery, and a 75% reduction in mortality rates."[49]

In another important study, Dr. Kory explained how Ivermectin was used prophylactically among a group of 1,195 health care workers over a 3-month period. There were *no infections* among the 788 workers that took only 12 mg of Ivermectin once a week. However, among the 407 in the control group that did not take it as a preventative, 58% became ill with COVID-19.[50]

Critics, such as the one in an article and cleverly (but somewhat misleadingly) edited video,[51] are quick to point out that in August 2021, Dr. Kory himself got infected with COVID while on his original protocol of taking Ivermectin only once per week. Critics claim this proves Ivermectin does not work, and mock him for claiming that anyone who took Ivermectin would not get sick. However, they have trouble accepting the fact that when Dr. Kory made the statement, that was true in his experience up to that time. Then as variants emerged, it is not surprising if a protocol or dosage had to be adjusted. The critics appear to ignore that need for adjustment to variants and the vast amount of other evidence of the drug's efficacy.

India's most populous state, Uttar Pradesh, gave Ivermectin to all of its 240 million people, both as a prophylactic and as early treatment. *Ivermectin basically eradicated COVID in that large state. 240 million people!* Their rapid response teams took it prophylactically for several months and none got sick, even working in the highest risk situations.[52] Dr. Bartlett says that India was also using Budesonide as a primary treatment for its 1.2 billion people.[53]

Other Data of Deaths and Hospitalizations Avoided

Doctors have estimated that **as many as 85% of the deaths attributed to COVID-19 could have been avoided by early treatment** with proven multi-drug protocols.[54] In Dr. Bartlett's interview cited earlier, he said he believes 90% of hospitalizations could have been avoided with Budesonide. One of the other physicians who has had great success in saving the lives of COVID patients is Dr. Ben Marble, who founded www.MyFreeDoctor.com, a tele-med service. Between the spring of 2020 and August 2022, he personally had treated over 15,000 COVID patients. He and his team have collectively delivered over 300,000 *free* doctor visits, about half of which were acute COVID. Since that time, only six of their patients have died.[55]

Dr. George Fareed, MD and Dr. Bryan Tyson, MD, are co-authors of the book *Overcoming the COVID Darkness: How Two Doctors Successfully Treated 7,000 Patients.* Their early treatment for those 7,000 patients resulted in only four hospitalizations and *no deaths*.[56]   One report about Ivermectin says:

> "In the WHO's summary of findings, they suddenly include data from seven studies, which combined show an 81% reduction in deaths [by using Ivermectin]."[57]

Yet the WHO continues *not* to recommend Budesonide, Ivermectin or HCQ as a treatment for COVID-19, all of which are on its list of "essential medicines." **Why not?**

If front-line health care workers and the general public had taken Ivermectin prophylactically or even in the hospital, as in the above studies, imagine how different "all things COVID" would likely have been.

A person does not have to be a doctor to see that there is something very wrong with this picture. The government is surely aware of such data. **Yet they refuse to approve any of the above drugs or protocols as a treatment for COVID-19.** Instead, they claim these drugs are dangerous and ineffective. In fact, Dr. Robert Malone, one of the original inventors of the mRNA technology platform, has stated as recently as July 2022 that in the FDA's latest EUA review of the COVID vaccines, it still maintains there are no effective treatments.[58] **Why?**

Why would they ignore the pleas of doctors who were having great success with early treatments using proven protocols and all of the data from all of the many studies? As far as the CDC and Anthony Fauci were concerned, there were no early treatments for COVID-19. **Doctors, does that sound rational to you?** It did not sound rational to Dr. Richard Urso, an ophthalmologist, drug design and treatment specialist and co-founder of the International Alliance of Physicians and Medical Scientists. He stated:

> "All of a sudden when the word COVID-19, coronavirus, came up, there was no treatment for inflammation, no treatment for respiratory compromise, no treatment for blood clotting. *How is that possible? It's completely absurd.*"[59]

The purposeful campaign to villainize early treatment was absolutely necessary or else an Emergency Use Authorization of a vaccine could not have been granted. Hence, all the major and social media, the medical boards, and the three letter agencies threatened and intimidated health care providers into not rendering early treatment. If you understand the "big picture" that COVID fits into, as explained in Part 4 of this book, you will know the even greater reason.

The Misleading "95% Effective" Claim

Another point that relates to whether or not the vaccines were even necessary is found in the context of claims that the "vaccines" were "95% effective." That claim was based on clinical trial data, and was repeatedly made in the major media, including by government officials. However, that figure is extremely misleading because it represents only the "relative risk reduction," or RRR, not the "absolute risk reduction" or ARR. "Absolute risk reduction (ARR) – also called risk difference (RD) – is the most useful way of presenting research results to help your decision-making."[60] In this case, there is a huge difference between the two measures. That is why FDA guidelines specifically say that the ARR should always be included in a manufacturer's application and information given to the public:

> "Patients are unduly influenced when risk information is presented using a relative risk approach; this can result in suboptimal decisions. Thus, an absolute risk format should be used." [61]

Pfizer did not do this, and the FDA apparently ignored the omission, in violation of its own guidelines.[62] People relied on this claim that the shots were "95% effective" in preventing infection. The ARR measured how many bad outcomes (i.e., COVID infections) would be prevented by getting the intervention (the shot). In other words, how many in the control group who got the placebos actually got COVID, over and above the number who got the real "vaccine" and still got COVID? In contrast, the RRR only measures the reduction between the ARR and the "relative risk," or the RR. The data in Table 6 below, from Pfizer's clinical trials, were used to make the 95% calculation.[63]

Table 6. Pfizer Clinical Trial data: the basis of their "95% effectiveness" claim

PFIZER Trials	Size of group	# who got COVID-19	# who got COVID, expressed as a %
Vaccinated	18,198	8	0.04%
Unvaxxed control group	18,325	162	0.88%

The ARR is the difference between the above two percentages: 0.88 – 0.04 = 0.84% ARR. The RRR is calculated as follows: 1 – (8/162) = .95062 or 95%.

In other words, Pfizer's own clinical trial data show that at that time, the **risk of getting COVID-19 without any inoculation was less than 1% (only 0.88%)! And those who received the shot reduced their risk from 0.88% to 0.04%. It is that reduction that the 95% figure represents.** Astoundingly, the benefit of getting the shot was almost nil in the first place, according to Pfizer's own clinical trial data.

The above data were among those on which Pfizer received EUA. If Pfizer's numbers are reasonably correct, those under 70 among the 0.88% who got COVID without the shots had an infection fatality rate of only 0.00003 to 0.005, based on the CDC's estimates from September 10, 2020 presented above. **Based on those data alone, why was a vaccine even necessary?**

There is reason to believe that the above Pfizer numbers may *not* be reasonably correct, and that the RRR may actually be much lower. Dr. Peter Doshi, an Associate Professor of Pharmaceutical Health Services Research in the School of Pharmacy at the University of Maryland, did an analysis of Pfizer clinical trial data.[64] He noted that the numbers of confirmed cases as shown in the above table (8 and 162) "were dwarfed by a category of disease called 'suspected covid-19'—those with symptomatic covid-19 that were not PCR confirmed." That information was in the "FDA Briefing Document" presented at the December 10, 2020 meeting of the FDA's VRBPAC (Vaccine and Related Biological Products Advisory Committee) at which Pfizer's EUA application was to be acted upon. That document showed "3,410 total cases of suspected, but unconfirmed covid-19 in the overall study population, 1594 occurred in the vaccine group vs. 1816 in the placebo group."[65] **Why is there such a large group of unconfirmed symptomatic cases? Why were they not counted?** We do not know, but according to Doshi, the information about this large group of suspected cases was not included in Pfizer's report or in its publication of clinical trial data in the *NEJM*. It was found only in the FDA report referred to above. **Were they trying to hide this information?**

Doshi stated that this large group of suspected-but-not-confirmed participants should not be ignored just because they lacked a positive PCR test. If all such cases had been included in the calculations, Doshi concluded: "A rough estimate of vaccine efficacy against developing COVID-

WAS A VACCINE EVEN NECESSARY?

19 symptoms, with or without a positive PCR test result, would be a relative risk reduction of 19% ... far below the 50% effectiveness threshold for authorization set by regulators." He further noted: "Even after removing cases occurring within 7 days of vaccination (409 on Pfizer's vaccine vs. 287 on placebo), which should include the majority of symptoms due to short-term vaccine reactogenicity, vaccine efficacy remains low: 29%." [66]

He acknowledged the difficulty posed by the fact that influenza-like illnesses can have a variety of causes, but without more data and the reason why these suspected cases were not included in the risk reduction calculations, Pfizer's 95% RRR is open to question. *Were none of the "suspected-but-not-confirmed" participants actually tested? If not, why not, since they were symptomatic? Could it be that Pfizer was manipulating how many in the "suspected-but-not-confirmed" group they would actually test in order to come up with an RRR of 95%?*

The Case and Death Numbers Were Grossly Inflated

It is well-established that both the number of COVID cases and deaths were grossly inflated. They both contributed to the *perception* of a dangerous pandemic. The PCR test was used to determine a "case," even though its inventor specifically said it could *not* be used to diagnose a disease because, he said, PCR is a *process*, *not* for diagnosis. [67] The FDA admits that they had to use "contrived samples" of the virus to develop the test in the first place, because they had no actual samples![68]

CDC's instruction sheets to labs say to run the test using a cycle threshold (Ct) of 40, and most US labs were running them at 37-40 Ct.[69] However, running the test over a Ct of 35 was found to result in a rate of false positives as high as 90%.[70] An international team of 22 experts who reviewed the original report that the COVID PCR test was based on said that **the false positive rate could have been as high as 97%.** [71] Even Dr. Fauci conceded that a Ct rate over 35 was meaningless, and the chances of it being "replication competent" [i.e., accurate] were "miniscule."[72] In July 2021, the CDC announced it was withdrawing the PCR test for COVID at the end of the year because it could not sufficiently distinguish between COVID and the flu![73] *For almost 2 years*, many tens of millions of "cases" were counted as COVID based on a deeply flawed test, and flu cases disappeared -- apparently into the COVID column.

COVID Deaths

The "COVID death" count was also grossly inflated. That was due in large part to a change in March 2020 in the CDC guidelines for reporting COVID-related deaths, as further explained in a Guidance document several days later. The change said to put COVID on the death certificate even "in cases where a definite diagnosis of COVID cannot be made."[74] That change resulted in far more deaths attributed to COVID than there should have been. *Might the fact that hospitals received significant financial remuneration for each case and death designated as COVID-19 also have added to the numbers for both cases and deaths?*

The CDC's website showed that **in 2020 *only 6% of "COVID death" numbers reported in the major media were actually deaths "from" COVID-19 alone.* For 2021 that number was only 5+%.**[75] The rest were people who died with multiple other health conditions or from other causes such as accidents, who may or may not have died "with" COVID but not "from" it.

A peer-reviewed paper written by a group of ten scientists, doctors and professors entitled "COVID-19 Data Collection, Comorbidity & Federal Law: A Historical Retrospective," was published October 12, 2020 in the journal *Science, Public Health Policy & the Law*.[76] It explains that prior to that March 2020 change, the CDC's death reporting guidelines had been in effect since 2003.-*Under those guidelines, only 6% of the "COVID deaths" in 2020 would have been counted as "COVID deaths."* That aligns exactly with the statements on the CDC website mentioned in the previous paragraph. That paper also revealed a history of "what appears to be manipulative data practices by the CDC" that violated federal law. It says the March 2020 change in death reporting did not go through the process required for proposed regulatory changes. That would make it invalid. But the damage it did cannot be undone.

The CDC has also admitted that its COVID death count had serious errors.[77] In March 2022, it reported that it had wrongly included more than 72,000 deaths as COVID deaths, allegedly due to a "coding error." It also had to reduce pediatric COVID deaths by 416 from its initial count, a reduction of about 24%. But again, the damage had already been done from the overly-inflated numbers. Alameda County in California had to reduce its death count by 25% in June 2021, "to comply with the state's definition

WAS A VACCINE EVEN NECESSARY?

of a COVID-19 death, which requires COVID-19 to be a direct or contributing factor or a situation in which it can't be ruled out."[78] ***Why were they not complying before? Was there a change in the definition there too? How many other counties may also have had these kinds of errors?***

If COVID-19 were as deadly as they claimed, this should have shown up as excess deaths in 2020 in the all-cause mortality data. *Does it? Technocracy News* reports that a professor at Johns Hopkins University "published a devastating exposé of hysterical pandemic exaggeration, which was dramatically 'un-published' shortly thereafter … [b]ecause it crushed the global narrative that COVID is driving up overall death numbers." That study showed no excess deaths between mid-March and mid-September 2020, even among the elderly.[79] That was the most critical period for determining if a vaccine was even needed or justified.

Other sources also confirm the lack of excess deaths. A group of 46 UK funeral directors all reported no increase in deaths during the "pandemic."[80] It was reported by a Canadian casket maker in July 2022 that they had expected an uptick in sales in 2020, due to what the public was being told about the lethality of COVID. However, he estimated that their business *actually dropped about 60% in 2020,* because people were locked down and not traveling or involved in their normal activities. They did not see an increase until after the vaccine rollout. He described the increase in their business in 2022 as "staggering," especially after the boosters started.[81]

Also, according to the American Council of Life Insurers, insurers paid out only 4,299,000 life insurance policies in 2020, compared to 4,776,000 in 2018 and 4,644,000 in 2012.[82] Even if there were excess deaths, *how many actually resulted **not** from COVID but from the hospital treatment protocols, consequences of the lockdowns, or data manipulation by the government?*

Compare that with the official narrative. We were all told that COVID was so deadly that we had to have lock downs, school closings, social distancing, mask mandates, a huge vaccine campaign, vaccine mandates and in some places, vaccine passports. We were told that vaccines were the only solution to end the crisis, that there was no treatment for COVID-19.

To sum up: if 1) 90-97% of the positive PCR tests were false; 2) only 6% of the deaths reported as COVID deaths were actually deaths from COVID; 3) most people's symptoms were no more serious than a seasonal flu; 4) the survival rate for most was over 99.4% in 2020 and 2021; 5) effective treatments were available; 6) the 95% effective claim only reduced the chances of infection from 0.88% to 0.04% (assuming Pfizer's numbers were accurate); and 7) it appears there was no excess death rate in 2020, *does that sound like a "dangerous pandemic" to you? Based on the above evidence, do you believe that a vaccine was even necessary?*

As stated earlier, if a vaccine was not even necessary, why has the medical industrial complex been so hell-bent on everyone getting these shots, plus who knows how many boosters?

Sadly, the evidence reveals that we can no longer trust those who have been entrusted with the responsibility to provide accurate and truthful information about matters of public health, even those involving life and death. Not anymore. Based on the government's and manufacturers' own documents, data and other evidence, *one theme that runs throughout the whole COVID story is this: our own government, Big Pharma, the major media, and others have been lying about "all things COVID" from the very beginning.* The destruction that COVID has wrought cannot be attributed only to bad policies, honest mistakes, incompetence or even greed – or even a virus. If I had the slightest doubt about that, I would not have bothered writing this book. If I were still practicing law and had a license at stake, I would stake my license and livelihood on it – just as many brave doctors, scientists and others have done who have risked everything by daring to contradict the official narrative.

---

[28] Toby Rogers, Ph.D., https://brownstone.org/articles/the-fdas-future-framework-for-covid-vaccines-is-reckless-plan/ (June 22, 2022)

[29] Dr. Michael Yeadon presentation, https://odysee.com/@Quasar:3/Mike-Yeadon-Testimony-for-the-Grand-Jury:9 (testimony date Feb. 4, 2022)

[30] Daniel Horowitz, https://www.theblaze.com/op-ed/horowitz-the-cdc-confirms-remarkably-low-coronavirus-death-rate-where-is-the-media (May 25, 2020)

[31] Daniel Horowitz, https://www.theblaze.com/conservative-review/horowitz-new-antibody-study-strong-evidence-lockdown-strategy-wrong-course (April 20, 2020)

[32] Anthony S. Fauci, M.D., H. Clifford Lane, M.D., and Robert R. Redfield, M.D., COVID-19 – Navigating the Uncharted, N Engl J Med 2020; 382:1268-1269 DOI: 10.1056/NEJMe2002387; https://www.nejm.org/doi/full/10.1056/NEJMe2002387

[33] https://web.archive.org/web/20201127224157/https://www.cdc.gov/coronavirus/2019-ncov/hcp/planning-scenarios.html

[34] https://willemvincken.wordpress.com/2022/02/05/the-covid-survival-rates-with-without-vaccine-no-differences/ (Feb. 5, 2022)

[35] Taylor Smith and Jack Lowenstein, https://www.winknews.com/2020/09/23/cdc-shows-covid-19-has-high-survival-rate-doctor-still-wants-to-see-precautions-taken/ (updated Sept. 26, 2020)

[36] Peter R. Breggin, MD & Ginger Ross Breggin, *COVID-19 and the Global Predators: We are the Prey* (2021), pp. 132-133

[37] Ibid., p. xiv.

[38] Bryan Fischer, "HCQ Is the Answer to COVID-19 – Don't Let Them Lie to You," https://www.afa.net/the-stand/culture/2020/07/hcq-is-the-answer-to-covid-19-don-t-let-them-lie-to-you/ (July 31, 2020)

[39] Dr. Meryl Nass, https://anthraxvaccine.blogspot.com/2020/05/hydroxychloroquine-keeping-you-updated.html (May 29, 2020)

[40] Donald C. Pompan, MD and Michael M. Jacobs, MD, MPH, https://www.thedesertreview.com/opinion/letters_to_editor/the-assault-against-early-treatment-for-covid-19-how-one-congressional-hearing-speaks-volumes-about/article_33425ff2-3593-11eb-b0d2-cf1365831d45.html (Dec. 3, 2020, updated April 16, 2021)

[41] Stella Immanuel, MD, *Let America Live*, pp. 4-6,40-49.

[42] Dr. Richard Bartlett interviewed by Scott McKay, March 1, 2022, https://www.onenewspage.com/video/20220302/14436777/Interview-with-Dr-Richard-Bartlett-Frontline-Doctors.htm

[43] https://budesonideworks.com/studies-reports/

[44] https://newcomz.wordpress.com/2021/05/23/Ivermectin-has-saved-a-lot-of-lives-from-covid-19-around-the-world/ (May 23, 2021)

[45] Id.

[46] https://covid19criticalcare.com/

[47] https://drpierrekory.com/about

[48] Dr. Pierre Kory testimony on effectiveness and safety of Ivermectin in Senate hearing of the Homeland Security & Governmental Affairs Committee, https://www.c-span.org/video/?c4930160/user-clip-dr-pierre-kory-senate-hearing-Ivermectin-100-cure-covid-19 (Dec. 8, 2020)

[49] https://newcomz.wordpress.com/2021/05/23/Ivermectin-has-saved-a-lot-of-lives-from-covid-19-around-the-world/ (May 23, 2021)

[50] Nadya Swart, https://www.biznews.com/health/2021/07/29/ivermectin-treatment (July 29, 2021)

[51] https://www.techarp.com/science/covid-19-dr-pierre-kory-ivermectin (Dec. 30, 2021)

[52] Rafael Castillo, MD, https://lifestyle.inquirer.net/389302/uttar-pradesh-is-Ivermectins-best-practice-success-story/ (Oct. 5, 2021)(last accessed April 29, 2022)

[53] Dr. Richard Bartlett interviewed by Scott McKay, March 2022, https://www.onenewspage.com/video/20220302/14436777/Interview-with-Dr-Richard-Bartlett-Frontline-Doctors.htm

[54] For example, Dr. Peter McCullough interviewed by Joe Rogan, https://www.thebiglogic.com/85-of-covid-deaths-couldve-been-avoided-with-early-treatment-dr-peter-mccullough/ (Dec, 2021)

[55] Correspondence between Sally Saxon and Dr. Ben Marble, Aug. 2022.

[56] Tyson, Brian; Fareed, George; Crawford, Mathew. *Overcoming the COVID Darkness: How Two Doctors Successfully Treated 7000 Patients* (p. 155). Brian Tyson, M.D. and George C. Fareed, M.D., Kindle Edition.

[57] https://newcomz.wordpress.com/2021/05/23/Ivermectin-has-saved-a-lot-of-lives-from-covid-19-around-the-world/ (May 23, 2021)

[58] Dr. Robert Malone, Dr. Pierre Kory and Dr. Richard Urso interviewed by Del Bigtree, https://thehighwire.com/videos/malone-urso-kory-stop-vaccinating/ (July 15, 2022)

[59] https://www.thethinkingconservative.com/increase-in-reactivated-viruses-following-covid-19-booster-shots-dr-richard-urso/ (April 30, 2022)

⁶⁰ https://www.ncbi.nlm.nih.gov/books/NBK63647/
⁶¹ https://www.fda.gov/media/81597/download p. 60
⁶² Dr. Ron Brown, https://trialsitenews.com/will-fda-mrna-vaccine-approval-ignore-the-elephant-not-in-the-room-ultra-low-absolute-risk-reductions/ (Aug. 10, 2021)
⁶³ Canadian COVID Care Alliance, "Relative vs Absolute Risk Reduction," https://rumble.com/vobcg5-relative-vs-absolute-risk-reduction.html (Oct. 27, 2021)
⁶⁴ Dr. Peter Doshi, https://blogs.bmj.com/bmj/2021/01/04/peter-doshi-pfizer-and-modernas-95-effective-vaccines-we-need-more-details-and-the-raw-data/ (Jan. 4, 2021, clarified in another post Feb.5, 2021).
⁶⁵ https://www.fda.gov/media/144245/download
⁶⁶ His calculations in the footnote to the *BMJ* article were as follows: 19% = 1 – (8+1594)/(162+1816); 29% = 1 – (8 + 1594 – 409)/(162 + 1816 – 287). Doshi "ignored denominators as they are similar between groups."
⁶⁷ Panel with Dr. Kary Mullis, "Kary Mullis Explains the PCR Test," https://www.youtube.com/watch?v=ZmZft4fXhQQ
⁶⁸ https://www.fda.gov/medical-devices/coronavirus-covid-19-and-medical-devices/sars-cov-2-reference-panel-comparative-data
⁶⁹ Stacey Lennox, https://web.archive.org/web/20210121211954/https://pjmedia.com/columns/stacey-lennox/2021/01/20/the-who-finally-updates-its-covid-19-testing-policy-1-hour-after-bidens-inauguration-n1398857 (Jan 20, 2021)
⁷⁰ Apoorva Mandavilli, "Your Coronavirus test is Positive. Maybe It Shouldn't Be," https://www.nytimes.com/2020/08/29/health/coronavirus-testing.html (Aug. 29, 2020, updated July 23, 021)
⁷¹ An International Consortium of Scientists, https://cormandrostenreview.com/report/ (Nov. 27, 2020)
⁷² Comments by Dr. Anthony Fauci, "This Week in Virology" Podcast, https://www.youtube.com/watch?v=a_Vy6fgaBPE&t=241s (July 16, 2020)
⁷³ https://www.cdc.gov/locs/2021/07-21-2021-lab-alert-Changes_CDC_RT-PCR_SARS-CoV-2_Testing_1.html
⁷⁴ https://www.cdc.gov/nchs/data/nvss/vsrg/vsrg03-508.pdf , p. 2; https://www.cdc.gov/nchs/data/nvss/coronavirus/Alert-2-New-ICD-code-introduced-for-COVID-19-deaths.pdf; Charles Creitz, https://www.foxnews.com/media/physician-blasts-cdc-coronavirus-death-count-guidelines (April 9, 2020)
⁷⁵ https://www.cdc.gov/nchs/nvss/vsrr/covid_weekly/index.htm (use www.archive.org for past weeks' data.)
⁷⁶ https://thecovidblog.com/2021/02/12/peer-reviewed-manuscript-concludes-that-cdc-massively-inflates-covid-19-case-and-death-numbers-with-creative-statistics/ (Feb. 12, 2021)
⁷⁷ https://www.dailywire.com/news/cdc-overreported-covid-19-deaths-by-more-than-70000 (March 23, 2022)
⁷⁸ Matt Boone, https://archive.ph/oe839#selection-2209.0-2233.229 (June 7, 2021)
⁷⁹ https://www.technocracy.news/johns-hopkins-u-s-death-rate-remains-normal-despite-covid-19/ (Nov. 30, 2020)
⁸⁰ https://stopworldcontrol.com/downloads/en/vaccines/vaccinereport.pdf, p. 25
⁸¹ Miranda Sellick, https://rairfoundation.com/coffins-for-children-ordered-in-bulk-first-time-in-over-30-years-exclusive-interview/ (July 14, 2022)
⁸² Darby Shaw, https://darbyshaw.substack.com/p/what-wheres-the-excess-mortality?s=r#_ftn3 (Jan. 10, 2022)

Chapter 5
Were the Emergency Use Requirements Met?

In 2020, and for subsequent FDA authorizations of the COVID vaccines for children and the early adult boosters, these experimental vaccines were released into the marketplace only for emergency use under federal law. They were not licensed or "approved" by the FDA. Although the FDA was reported to have "fully approved" the Pfizer "vaccine" on August 23, 2021, there is much confusion as to what the FDA's action actually amounted to. However, the details of that issue are not addressed in this book. Regardless of what Pfizer and the FDA intended the public to believe about that action, what we do know is this: the original formulations, as well as the current boosters for adults and the shots authorized for children that are currently being administered (as of the fall of 2022) are under Emergency Use Authorization (EUA). They have not been FDA "approved" or licensed.

Federal law has four criteria for a drug to qualify for EUA, and if even one of these criteria is not met, EUA cannot be granted *or maintained*. [83]

- The ... agent referred to in the March 27, 2020, EUA declaration by the Secretary of HHS (SARS-CoV-2) can cause a serious or life-threatening disease or condition. (i.e., there must be an "emergency.")
- Based on the totality of scientific evidence available, including data from adequate and well-controlled trials, if available, it is reasonable to believe that the product may be effective to prevent, diagnose, or treat such serious or life-threatening disease or condition...
- The known and potential benefits of the product, when used to diagnose, prevent, or treat the identified serious or life-threatening disease or condition, outweigh the known and potential risks of the product.
- There is no adequate, approved, and available alternative to the product for diagnosing, preventing, or treating the disease or condition.

Based on strong and substantial evidence, it appears that the COVID shots failed to meet these criteria. Keep them in mind as you read through the book, and consider whether you think each one has been continually met, based on clinical trial results and *at all times since.* If even one of the four were not met, either initially or at any time since, that would render the EUA invalid and the shots should be halted. For example, *has there really been an ongoing public health emergency the entire time since early 2020 until today, in late 2022?* Even if there is still an official government *declaration* of an emergency, which is required for an EUA to be granted or maintained, **does an "emergency" really still exist at this point in time, especially when effective treatments are available?** *Or is the government maintaining and renewing emergency declarations only to justify the continuation of the shots, regardless of the degree of any actual threat?*

Also, note that the standard for efficacy is much lower for EUA than for FDA "licensure approval." EUA requires only that the totality of evidence shows that "it is *reasonable to believe* that the product *may be* effective." That is less than an "**is** effective" standard. But continual representations have been made that the COVID shots "*are* safe and effective," as though the higher standard had been met. Therefore, their claims must be judged by that higher standard.

There is also an issue as to whether or not the words "safe and effective" may legally be used to describe and promote an *unlicensed, experimental* product, since "safe and effective" is a "term of art" used by the FDA for *licensed* products.[84] Dr. Meryl Nass, MD, gave testimony on that point in a state government committee hearing.[85] *Did the government violate its own regulations or guidelines in using these words?* Regulatory agencies have specific rules about what kinds of representations and claims *may and may not be made* about a product. For example, if a company or spokesperson states that its product "will cure cancer," a cease-and-desist demand would surely follow.

This is not a minor issue, since billions of people around the world relied heavily on the claim of "safe and effective" in making their decision to get the shots. However, because it relates more to how the shots have been represented rather than to matters that directly affect their safety or effectiveness, it is not addressed in detail here. The significance of the issue for purposes of this book is whether or not it was a fraudulent misrepresentation that led people to take certain action they otherwise would not have taken, and then caused harm.

WERE THE EMERGENCY USE REQUIREMENTS MET?

- *How many people do you think would have chosen to get the shots if the claim of "safe and effective" had not been endlessly repeated by the medical industrial complex?*

- *What do you think the response would have been if it had been endlessly represented that these shots are experimental, have not been licensed and approved by the FDA and have not undergone long-term testing in humans?*

- *Has the government violated any of its own regulations or guidelines by allowing and using the words "safe and effective" to describe an unlicensed, experimental EUA product?*

---

[83] The criteria established by the U.S. HHS Section 564 of the Federal Food, Drug, and Cosmetic Act, summarized in an FDA document entitled "Guidance for Industry and Other Stakeholders: Emergency Use Authorization of Medical Products and Related Authorities" (March 31, 2022), https://www.fda.gov/media/142749/download.

[84] https://www.fda.gov/science-research/risk-communication/fdas-risk-communication-research-agenda;

[85] Meryl Nass, MD, Testimony, Maine Health and Human Services Committee, Jan. 11,2022, https://legislature.maine.gov/testimony/resources/HHS20220111NASS1328629 41356715133.pdf

Chapter 6
Why Many Have Not Heard This Information Before: *Reason #1*

*"To learn who rules over you,
simply find out who you are not allowed to criticize."*

Voltaire

This book is a challenge to many in the health care community to at least question whether what they have been told is really true. It seems inescapable, especially for those on the frontlines, that there are many things about "all things COVID" that just do not seem right. If you feel that way, and have experienced some degree of "cognitive dissonance" between what you have experienced and what you have been told, this book will help resolve that. Cognitive dissonance has been defined as "the mental discomfort that results from holding two conflicting beliefs, values, or attitudes."[86]

There are at least 3 main reasons why even the medical community has not been told the information that is reported in this book. The first will be shared now in Part 1. The other two will be revealed in later parts of the book.

Reason #1: Massive Censorship and Propaganda. As stated in the Declaration of the Global COVID Summit, a group of 17,000 physicians and medical scientists:

> **"The medical community has denied patients the fundamental human right to provide true informed consent for the experimental COVID-19 injections.** Our patients are also blocked from obtaining the information necessary to understand risks and benefits of vaccines, and their alternatives, due to widespread censorship and propaganda spread by governments, public health officials and media." [87]

WHY MANY HAVE NOT HEARD BEFORE: REASON #1

Dr. Robert Malone, one of the co-founders of this group has further commented on this:

> "We have also been living through the most massive, globally coordinated propaganda and censorship campaign in the history of the human race. All major mass media and the social media technology companies have coordinated to stifle and suppress any discussion of the risks of the genetic vaccines AND/OR alternative early treatments…
>
> "All opportunities for the victims to have become self-informed about the potential risks have been methodically erased from both the internet and public awareness by an international corrupt cabal operating under the flag of the 'Trusted News Initiative.'" [88]

The "Trusted News Initiative" refers to a worldwide effort to standardize and control the news through the corporate media and to alert each other to what they consider to be "disinformation." That would include topics such as COVID to ensure that anything contrary to their approved messaging is not published.[89] The Vaccine Safety Research Foundation has made an excellent 4-minute eye-opening video explaining more about this Initiative and all of the major media networks and outlets who are involved in it.[90] According to that video, the TNI uses algorithms to identify anti-vaccine content to be censored, while it floods the media with repetitive pro-vaccine messages. It also stigmatizes the unvaccinated in an attempt to create division and promote vaccine "compliance." It appears that the Trusted News Initiative cannot be trusted to provide the true and objective information that people need to make their own decisions. They only report what they want people to hear. ***Why are they so afraid of allowing people to think for themselves?***

Malone expounds further about those pushing the government narrative, many of whom he has known and worked with for decades:

> "They have been lying and lying and lying and lying. There are multiple layers of fraud going on…They're trying to get away with the fact that there were multiple misrepresentations that this vaccine could get us to herd immunity… The lies keep coming. They don't stop. They don't care." [91]

Some of the documentary evidence of the close coordination between government and social media companies that Malone referred to in censoring COVID information contrary to the official narrative was released in July 2022 as a result of a lawsuit against the CDC. The case was brought by a nonprofit organization, America First Legal, which described the documents as "the tip of the iceberg," showing coordination between government and Big Tech on social media platforms. [92]

One of the collaborating authors on this book, Dr. James A. Thorp, was the lead author of a paper entitled "Patient Betrayal: The Corruption of Healthcare, Informed Consent and the Physician-Patient Relationship." That report discussed how the "governing bodies of healthcare professionals have banded together in cartel-like fashion" threatening to destroy the livelihood of health care providers whom those bodies claim are spreading "misinformation." [93] That terminology, he says, describes anything that would tend to create "vaccine hesitancy," and is used to "discredit alternative views and seeks to prevent honest and truthful communication" between patients and their providers.

Yale Professor Dr. Harvey Risch, MD, explains that "censorship exists when the party that does the censoring cannot defend that position." [94] *If you believe that the vaccines are safe and effective, would you be able to defend that position with solid evidence?*

Retired neurosurgeon Dr. Russell Blaylock, MD, has written a blistering article explaining what is behind the censorship and demonization of highly respected physicians who have been saving countless lives with various multi-drug protocols and speaking out about the dangers of the COVID shots. He explains that it is the control of the pharmaceutical companies over the health care industry, including the major medical journals that rely on them for revenue. Even worse, he exposes that "Proven fraudulent 'ghostwritten' articles sponsored by pharmaceutical giants have appeared regularly in top clinical journals ... never to be removed despite proven scientific abuse and manipulation of data." [95]

One well-known example of this is the infamous paper by a lead author from Harvard published in *The Lancet* that Dr. James Thorp says consisted of "completely fraudulent data" that was not just manipulated — it was "completely falsified for the specific political purpose of doing a 'hatchet job' on hydroxychloroquine." This drug has an 85-year safety record and

WHY MANY HAVE NOT HEARD BEFORE: REASON #1

a safety profile better than that of aspirin or acetaminophen. But *The Lancet's* deception was exposed, and it was forced it to retract the paper.[96]

Blaylock also explains that these same pharmaceutical companies essentially control the major media as well, since about 70% of "all news advertising" revenues in the U.S. come from them. How many times have we heard and seen on the major networks' news shows: "Brought to you by Pfizer"? As Blaylock also points out, those companies spend about $20 billion/year, or 68% of their medical marketing budget, on persuading medical professionals to prescribe their products.

Another example that should raise questions about the motives and objectives of high government officials is found in an email dated October 8, 2020 from then NIH Director Francis Collins to Dr. Anthony Fauci.[97] Collins was concerned about the Great Barrington Declaration,[98] a document signed by tens of thousands of doctors, public health scientists and others. It expressed concerns about the government's COVID policies, and suggested a better approach to the crisis. The email to Fauci says:

> "See https://gbdeclaration.org/ This proposal from the three fringe epidemiologists who met with the Secretary seems to be getting a lot of attention – and even a co-signature from Nobel Prize winner Mike Leavitt at Stanford. ***There needs to be a quick and devastating published takedown of its premises.*** I don't see anything like that on line yet – is it underway?" (emphasis added)

Think about that: ***a high government official advocating "a quick and devastating published take down"*** of a good faith solution proposed by experienced physicians seeking to end a national crisis. Collins then demeans the three doctors by calling them "fringe epidemiologists." One of those alleged "fringe" doctors is a Professor of Medicine at Harvard, another is a Professor of Medicine at Stanford, and the other is a Professor at Oxford. And do not forget the Nobel Prize winner. ***Why would officials have such a condescending attitude towards thousands of well-meaning, caring doctors expressing legitimate concerns and suggesting practical solutions?***

Also beware of the so-called "fact-checkers." Most of them are run or funded by those whose facts they are checking or those who have a vested interest in promoting the official "safe and effective" narrative. To them, anything that is contrary to the official narrative is "dis- or misinformation." The evidence be damned. ***Who then are the real spreaders of "misinformation"?***

Even internet searches on Google and other search engines have played a role in keeping people from finding important information that contradicts the official narrative. As reported in *The Gateway Pundit*, one of the medical industrial complex's biggest targets of alleged "misinformation":

> "Google ostensibly manipulated its search engine results and algorithm to bury the facts about mRNA technology as YouTube and every major tech giant purged users from their platforms for diverging even an iota from the World Health Organization's speech parameters, setting a precedent that deteriorates the First Amendment."[99]

Despite the massive censorship, lies and coverups by the major media, as of late summer 2022 some media figures have finally started to acknowledge and discuss the devastation caused by the COVID shots. It remains to be seen whether this is because the damage from the shots has become too obvious to continue ignoring, or whether it signifies a shift that has been long in coming in the major media's reporting of the truth.

In the last half of 2022, Tucker Carlson on the FOX Network started reporting on the problems the shots have been creating in the body, such as suppressing the immune system, and the fact that the death rates have been soaring worldwide. Soon afterwards, talk show host Dan Bongino publicly shared that getting the COVID shots was the biggest mistake and biggest regret of his life, especially after listening to Carlson's report.[100]

On a podcast episode in August 2022, former FOX News anchor Megyn Kelly gave a scathing rebuke of Anthony Fauci for all of his lies and the enormous damage he has done to America in his handling of COVID.[101] Also in August 2022, Wayne Allyn Root wrote an article[102] about Carlson's reporting on these issues and Bongino's comments, noting how some of the major media figures seem to have been "waking up" to what he and many others had been reporting for a year and a half. He suggested there may be political reasons for that, but whatever the reasons, it is still a significant shift.

WHY MANY HAVE NOT HEARD BEFORE: REASON #1

However, as stated earlier, even if the COVID vaccines have been stopped by the time you are reading this, the information in this book is still critical for the health care community and others because the lessons to be learned from these shots go far beyond "all things COVID."

Reason #2 why many have not heard much of the information in this report before will explain the "why" behind all of the censorship and propaganda. Reason #3 will explain the even bigger "why" behind the first two reasons. If everyone had been aware of even one of these reasons or just some of the information in this book before the vaccine rollout, it is highly doubtful that the vast majority of people would have chosen to get the COVID shots.

Whose report will you believe? The official-narrative that the COVID-19 vaccines are "safe and effective," as well as necessary? Or, *will you believe the evidence presented by countless thousands of doctors, other health care professionals, scientists, and experts worldwide who have risked everything by contradicting that narrative and warning the public of what they believe are great dangers?* Let us now jump into the fray in Part 2.

Part 2 presents substantial evidence of the degree and nature of harm caused by these shots, not just from government data, but from several other reliable sources with highly relevant information. Here are some of the questions to which you will find answers in Part 2:

What picture does data in the Vaccine Adverse Event Reporting System (VAERS) paint?

How has the government's response to the adverse event and death data in VAERS been so drastically different for COVID-19 vaccines than for all other vaccines and even drugs in general?

How have the data concerning the effects of the vaccines on pregnant women been manipulated?

How has the U.S. military been decimated by the COVID shots, especially because of the mandates?

Why have so many physicians and professional medical coalitions adamantly warned that these shots should not be given to children?

What are the dangers of the spike protein that we were not warned about?

How are the vaccines damaging the natural immune system?

— *Why are many pharmaceutical company employees concerned about these shots and why have many chosen not to get them?*

What is revealed in Pfizer's and Moderna's documents that raises serious concerns about safety?

---

[86] Kendra Cherry, https://www.verywellmind.com/what-is-cognitive-dissonance-2795012 (July 29, 2022)

[87] www.GlobalCOVIDSummit.org

[88] Dr. Robert Malone, "What if the largest experiment on human beings in history is a failure?" https://rwmalonemd.substack.com/p/what-if-the-largest-experiment-on (Jan. 2, 2022).

[89] https://expose-news.com/2021/08/29/the-trusted-news-initiative-a-bbc-led-organisation-censoring-public-health-experts-who-oppose-the-official-narrative-on-covid-19/ (Aug. 29, 2021)

[90] https://odysee.com/@VSRF:d/Vaccine-Safety-Research-Foundation-TNI:e

[91] Dr. Robert Malone, Dr. Pierre Kory and Dr. Richard Urso interviewed by Del Bigtree, https://thehighwire.com/videos/malone-urso-kory-stop-vaccinating/ (July 15, 2022) (starting around the 16:35 mark)

[92] https://greenmedinfo.com/blog/revealed-documents-show-collusion-between-cdc-and-big-tech (July 28, 2022)

[93] Thorp JA, Renz T, Northrup, C, Lively C, Breggin P, Bartlett R, et al. Patient Betrayal: The Corruption of Healthcare, Informed Consent and the Physician-Patient Relationship. G Med Sci. 2022; 3(1): 046-069. https://www.doi.org/10.46766/thegms.medethics.22021403

[94] Dr. Harvey Risch interviewed by Clay & Buck, https://www.clayandbuck.com/yale-epidemiologist-dr-harvey-risch-on-how-to-treat-covid/ (Sept. 27, 2001)

[95] Blaylock RL. COVID UPDATE: What is the truth?. Surg Neurol Int 22-Apr-2022;13:167. Available from: https://surgicalneurologyint.com/surgicalint-articles/covid-update-what-is-the-truth/

[96] Thorp JA, Renz T, Northrup, C, Lively C, Breggin P, Bartlett R, et al. Patient Betrayal: The Corruption of Healthcare, Informed Consent and the Physician-Patient Relationship. G Med Sci. 2022; 3(1): 046-069. https://www.doi.org/10.46766/thegms.medethics.22021403

[97] Paul Sacca, https://www.theblaze.com/news/fauci-email-francis-collins-great-barrington-declaration (Dec. 18, 2021)

[98] https://gbdeclaration.org/

[99] Alicia Powe, https://www.thegatewaypundit.com/2022/08/dan-bongino-reveals-getting-covid-vaccinated-greatest-regret-life/ (Aug. 23, 2022)

[100] Id.

[101] Chris Pandolfo, https://www.theblaze.com/news/megyn-kelly-anthony-fauci-take-down (Aug. 26, 2022).

[102] Wayne Allyn Root, https://www.thegatewaypundit.com/2022/08/wayne-root-blame-covid-vaccine-disaster-coverup-hint-not-president-donald-j-trump/ (Aug. 28, 2022)

PART 2

THE DANGERS AND GREAT HARM CAUSED BY THE SHOTS

"Find out just what any people will quietly submit to and you have the exact measure of the injustice and wrong which will be imposed on them."

Frederick Douglass
Social reformer, abolitionist, orator, writer and statesman

ACCESS TO HYPERLINKS *of* ONLINE REFERENCES

For easy access to hyperlinks for all of the online references cited in this book, use the QR code on the left or the "Endnotes Hyperlinks" button at www.SallySaxon.com.

Chapter 7
The "Most Dangerous Medicinal Product in History"

"Few men are willing to brave the disapproval of their fellows, the censure of their colleagues, the wrath of their society. Moral courage is a rarer commodity than bravery in battle or great intelligence. Yet it is the one essential, vital quality for those who seek to change a world which yields most painfully to change."[103]

Robert F. Kennedy
Former U.S. Attorney General, U.S. Senator and U.S. Presidential candidate

Initial questions:

- How can a vaccine be said to be "safe and effective" over the long term with only a few months of clinical trial data and NO long-term studies?
- If you believe that the COVID vaccines are safe, even without any data or knowledge of long-term effects, what scientific evidence is your belief based on?

Part 2 presents more extensive data, expert analyses and other information showing that the COVID vaccines are not only ***not*** safe and effective, but are actually dangerous and potentially extremely harmful, as the alleged "misinformation spreaders" have been warning about. It also summarizes and provides information about the mechanisms of injury caused by the shots; a comparison with the response to adverse reactions to the 1976 Swine flu vaccine; and the effects of the vaccines on pregnant women, the military, and those over 65. This part also discusses why countless thousands of doctors all over the world adamantly oppose giving these shots to children. Other issues include the dangers of the spike protein; the destructive impact of the COVID vaccines on the immune system; and the extreme discrepancies in the safety profiles between batches coming from the same manufacturer. Other key evidence revealing major problems is presented from Pfizer and Moderna documents. This part also provides other important safety-related information from former pharmaceutical company employees who have inside knowledge about the manufacturing process.

The COVID-19 "vaccines" are the "most dangerous biological medicinal product rollout in human history." [104]

That is a statement by Dr. Peter McCullough, MD, MPH, a renowned internist, cardiologist and epidemiologist, and a former Professor of Medicine. His conclusion is supported by many thousands of other doctors and medical scientists worldwide, as evidenced by Declarations of several groups representing tens of thousands of such professionals.[105] He is the most published doctor in his field in history, has been editor of a major journal in cardiovascular medicine, former editor of another journal, and was president of a major medical society for five years. When COVID broke out, he devoted all of his academic efforts to this topic. He has an academic medicine practice and spends about half of his time treating patients.

Dr. McCullough has been one of the most outspoken critics of the government's "no early treatment" policy and other hospital protocols. Like many other doctors, he has successfully treated and consulted on behalf of thousands of COVID patients with early treatment using a combination of drugs, including ones the CDC and FDA have suppressed and labelled as dangerous and ineffective. He also co-authored a best-selling book, *The Courage to Face COVID-19: Preventing Hospitalization and Death While Battling the Bio-Pharmaceutical Complex,* published in May 2022. It chronicles his journey to prevent as many COVID hospitalizations and deaths as possible, and his success in doing so.

When someone with his credentials makes a statement like the one above, should we not all pay attention? His 19-minute testimony at a Texas State Senate hearing explains why we should.[106] He led a team that was the first to publish a comprehensive outpatient COVID treatment protocol for doctors, entitled "Pathophysiological Basis and Rationale for Early Outpatient Treatment of SARS-CoV-2 Infection." It appeared in the August 2020 *American Journal of Medicine.*[107]

If anyone should enthusiastically support the continued administration of the COVID vaccines, you would think it would be Dr. Robert Malone,

MD. He is a vaccinologist and one of the original inventors of the mRNA platform used in the Pfizer and Moderna COVID shots. He received his first dose of the Moderna shot in April 2021, "long before the FOIA Japanese pre-clinical trial data that had so many red-flags and irregularities, long before we learned of all the issues with the clinical trials, and long before the VAERS and adverse events began to be known." [108] After almost dying following his second dose, he said: "I could never imagine that clinical data would be corrupted and even falsified - as we now know it was." He has since become one of the most vocal opponents of these injections, especially for children.

Doctors McCullough and Malone both realized early on after the vaccine rollout that something was not right about these shots, but it has taken many others much more time. This book and others addressing these issues are only necessary as there are many others who have yet to see the data and other important information such as that provided here.

Another physician who has changed his thinking about this debate is UK cardiologist Dr. Aseem Malhotra. In September 2022 he published a paper entitled "Curing the pandemic of misinformation on COVID-19 mRNA vaccines through real evidence-based medicine - Part 1." [109] He received the 2-dose primary series of the COVID shots shortly after the rollout, and publicly promoted the shots for quite a while based on what the health care community was being told about their safety and effectiveness. However, his own father, also a physician in excellent health, unexpectedly suffered cardiac arrest and died six months following his own COVID vaccinations. What Malhotra found "particularly shocking and inexplicable" about his father's death was that two of his major arteries showed severe blockages, one 90% and another 75%. After doing much research himself, he said:

> "I have slowly and reluctantly concluded contrary to my own initial dogmatic beliefs, Pfizer's mRNA vaccine is far from being as safe and effective as we once thought."

In July 2022, Dr. Brian Lenzkes, MD read reports that three young physicians at hospitals in Mississauga (Ontario, Canada) all died within a 3-day period just days after their 4th COVID shot. A fourth physician who worked nearby died while out for a run. After reading that news, he tweeted on July 15, 2022: "We are past the point of being able to walk away and say 'That is strange' to ourselves and walk on." He asks: *"How many more 'coincidences' will people accept? These shots need to be pulled."*[110]

Shortly after that tweet, three more Canadian doctors died following COVID shots, bringing the total to seven within two weeks.[111] None of these were elderly doctors. One was a triathlete and another was a marathon runner. The latest one was only 26 years old.

On August 28, 2022, it was reported that the Canadian doctors who have been dying since 2021 are much younger than in previous years.[112] According to the Canadian Medical Association data, the vast majority of Canadian doctors who died in 2019 and 2020 were elderly, mostly age 80 or older. Very few were younger than 60.[113] The CMA listed 246 deaths in 2020, and 393 in 2021. In 2020, before the vaccine rollout started, the death rate among Canadian doctors under 50 years of age was only about 6 per year.[114] However, after the latest mandated COVID booster, *6 doctors under 50 died within only 15 days!* That was calculated to represent 23X more deaths, or a 2,300% increase in all-cause mortality of Canadian doctors under 50 compared with the pre-rollout 2020 data.[115]

This book is to help health care professionals answer Dr. Lenzkes' question for themselves: ***how many more "coincidences" will you accept of many relatively healthy people dropping dead for no apparent reason very soon after receiving a COVID shot?*** Those who believe the shots are safe and effective usually base their opinion on what they have been told by the medical industrial complex. ***But do they know what they are NOT being told, and WHY?*** Part 1 has already revealed the massive coordinated campaign of lies and censorship of all those who dare to contradict the official narrative. As you continue reading through this book, the "whys" behind the lies and censorship will become increasingly clear.

Safety Concerns of Former Pharmaceutical Company Employees

Before more safety data and information is presented, the comments of two former pharmaceutical company employees will help to set the stage. They exemplify the concerns of unvaccinated persons all over the world. One was also speaking on behalf of himself and co-workers at Syneos Health, a large pharmaceutical company that employs representatives for various Johnson & Johnson drugs (though not for the COVID vaccines). They were fired for refusing the shots.[116] One employee said:

> "'A lot of us were questioning the shots because they didn't go through the proper safety and efficacy studies that are traditionally required for all medications . . . For there not to be safety and efficacy data with these COVID shots, many of us wanted to wait' ... 'The government said do this; it is in your best interest and you can go back to normal,' a former employee said. 'As time has gone on, we've seen, obviously, these are not actual vaccines that inoculate you and give you immunity. And there are a lot of reports of—and people that we know personally—who have been injured from these shots, so there's a good percentage of us that never got them. As data continued to come in, we were not going to get them..."

Another employee said it is "a matter of not living in fear," because so many people were living in fear "through what the media is telling them, and it's just unfortunate that more people don't actually do some research." That employee said:

> "'I know that COVID has taken people's lives just like the flu has, and pneumonia, and other viruses. But I'm not going to inject myself with something that has no long-term data. I'm not comfortable being an experiment for these pharmaceutical companies, and COVID has such a high percentage of survival rate that there's no need for me to.'"

Mechanisms of Injury from the COVID-19 Shots

Several mechanisms of injury from the COVID shots have been identified. Dr. Sherri Tenpenny, MD has listed more than 40 of them and has broken them down into 4 main groups:[117] 1) acute reactions; 2) illness/damage caused by the spike protein; 3) illness/damage caused by the anti-S-antibody; and 4) illness/damage caused to the immune system.

An excellent article about various mechanisms of injury is *"The Many Ways the COVID Vaccines May Harm Your Health"* by Dr. Joseph Mercola. It is based on his May 2022 interview with Dr. Stephanie Seneff (of MIT's Computer Science and Artificial Intelligence Lab) and Dr. Judy Mikovits. Dr. Mikovits says the various mechanisms "have synergistic effects when it comes to dysregulating …immune systems. 'It's just an explosion of a nightmare of crippling every area of your immune response.'" [118] That same article links to the interview transcript and an excellent report co-authored by Seneff entitled "Worse Than the Disease: Reviewing Some Possible Unintended Consequences of mRNA Vaccines Against COVID-19." [119]

Dr. James A. Thorp, an Ob-Gyn and maternal fetal specialist and a collaborating author of this book, has presented various mechanisms of injury with respect to pregnant women and women of reproductive age in a peer-reviewed medical journal paper entitled "Patient Betrayal: The Corruption of Healthcare, Informed Consent and the Physician-Patient Relationship." [120] Thorp focuses on three major etiopathophysiological mechanisms, including a dramatic vaccine-induced inflammatory effect, the adverse effects from the spike protein and the major damage done to the immune system, including the formation of auto-immune diseases.

In April of 2022, Thorp reviewed 1,366 peer-reviewed studies, and published his findings documenting severe morbidities and mortalities after the COVID-19 shots, with a hyperlink to a table of all of the studies organized by topic.[121] He estimates that as of early September 2022, there were almost 2,000 such studies. In the 32-year history of the Vaccine Adverse Event Reporting System (VAERS), no other vaccine has generated more than 50 such publications, according to Thorp. That is a factor of nearly 40 to 1. There is another similar list that includes 1,250 such papers.[122] *What does that suggest to you about the serious effects of the COVID shots?*

Doctors: are you looking for and recognizing vaccine-related injuries in your practice? Or are you attributing them to COVID or another cause, or even listing the cause as "unknown?

---

[103] One of Kennedy's statements quoted at his funeral service, June, 1968, http://www.tedkennedy.org/ownwords/event/eulogy.html

[104] Quoted in https://naturalnews.com/2021-12-25-covid-vaccines-most-dangerous-biological-product-peter-mccullough.html (Dec. 23, 2021)

[105] For example, www.GlobalCOVIDSummit.org representing 17,000 physicians and medical scientists.

[106] Dr. McCullough testimony, https://www.fulcrum7.com/blog/2021/8/13/a-closer-look-at-dr-peter-mccullough

[107] McCullough PA, Kelly RJ, Ruocco G, et al. Pathophysiological Basis and Rationale for Early Outpatient Treatment of SARS-CoV-2 (COVID-19) Infection. *Am J Med.* 2021;134(1):16-22. doi:10.1016/j.amjmed.2020.07.003; https://www.ncbi.nlm.nih.gov/pmc/articles/PMC7410805/

[108] https://rwmalonemd.substack.com/p/how-bad-is-my-batch?s=r

[109] Malhotra, A. Curing the pandemic of misinformation on COVID-19 mRNA vaccines through real evidence-based medicine - Part 1. Journal of Insulin Resistance | Vol 5, No 1 | a71 | DOI: https://doi.org/10.4102/jir.v5i1.71. https://insulinresistance.org/index.php/jir/article/view/71

[110] Reported by Steve Kirsch, https://stevekirsch.substack.com/p/will-physicians-ever-speak-out (July 23, 2022)

[111] Jim Hoft, https://www.thegatewaypundit.com/2022/08/26-year-old-neurosurgeon-dies-july-making-seven-canadian-doctors-die-two-weeks/ (Aug. 15, 2022)

[112] Steve Kirsch, https://stevekirsch.substack.com/p/over-30-deaths-of-young-healthy-canadian (Aug, 28, 2022)

[113] https://www.cma.ca/memoriam

[114] Steve Kirsch, https://stevekirsch.substack.com/p/doctors-in-canada-are-dying-at-a (Aug. 30, 2022)

[115] Id.

[116] Beth Brelje, https://www.theepochtimes.com/fired-pharmaceutical-workers-explain-why-they-didnt-get-covid-19-shots_4255408.html (Feb. 3, 2022)

[117] Dr. Sherri Tenpenny, *20 Mechanisms of Injury: How COVID 19 Injections Can Make You Sick... Even Kill You (2021),* and *20 More Mechanisms of Injury (2021),* available at www.DrTenpenny.com

[118] Dr. Joseph Mercola, https://www.theepochtimes.com/the-many-ways-in-which-covid-vaccines-may-harm-your-health_4441044.html?utm_source=ai&utm_medium=search (May 2, 2022)

[119] S. Seneff, S., G. Nigh, *International Journal of Vaccine Theory, Practice and Research* 2(1), May 10, 2021 (updated June 2021), https://ijvtpr.com/index.php/IJVTPR/article/view/23/139

[120] Thorp JA, Renz T, Northrup, C, Lively C, Breggin P, Bartlett R, et al. Patient Betrayal: The Corruption of Healthcare, Informed Consent and the Physician-Patient Relationship. G Med Sci. 2022; 3(1): 046-069, https://www.doi.org/10.46766/thegms.medethics.22021403, p. 9

[121] Hyperlink to 1,366 references for COVID-19 vaccine associated complications: https://www.thegms.co/publichealth/pubheal-rw-22042302-references.pdf

[122] https://react19.org/1250-covid-vaccine-reports/

Chapter 8
VAERS, V-Safe and Regulatory Agency Failures

Two of the CDC's vaccine safety monitoring systems are VAERS and V-Safe. VAERS was designed to be the government's "early warning" system, to warn of possible dangers once a vaccine has been rolled out. V-Safe is a phone app program which vaccinated persons could enroll in to report information about their condition following their COVID shots.

The COVID vaccine data have been sending many warning signals of significant adverse reactions to the shots since shortly after the rollout. But the warnings have gone unheeded and even denied. In the past, such as with respect to the swine flu and rotavirus vaccines, when certain numbers of injuries and deaths were reported after people took certain drugs, the government paused to investigate or stopped the vaccine campaign.

However, in the case of the COVID shots, instead of pausing or stopping the campaign, the government doubled-down and imposed mandates. It has even authorized the shots for children as young as 6 months old and continues to promote them as safe and effective. It has done so despite the pleas of many doctors, scientists, attorneys, and other experts all over the world to stop administering these shots because of the great damage they have wrought. *Why would the government do that?*

CDC Admissions of Withholding of Data, Failing to Monitor VAERS and False Reporting

On February 20, 2022, in an article entitled "The C.D.C. Isn't Publishing Large Portions of the Covid Data It Collects," the *New York Times* reported: *"Two full years into the pandemic, the agency leading the country's response to the public health emergency has published only a tiny fraction of the data it has collected, several people familiar with the data said."* One reason given by a CDC spokesperson for not releasing the data was that it might be misinterpreted. *Does the CDC think that health care professionals are not smart enough to interpret the data? Or might they be afraid that the alleged "misinformation spreaders" might expose the fact that the government's own data seriously undermine their official narrative?* Another reason given was that they needed to make sure the data was accurate. *How much more time do they need?* VAERS is supposed to be an "early warning system." *How can it provide early warnings if the data are delayed for many months or more than a year?*

Another problem is that the CDC has been continually claiming that the COVID vaccines have been subject to the "most intense safety monitoring program in U.S. history."[123] However, a recent admission reveals that not to be true. The CDC's own *Briefing Document* on procedures for monitoring VAERS for safety signals states that it "will perform PRR data mining on a weekly basis or as needed."[124] According to Josh Guetzkow, PhD, a senior lecturer in the Department of Sociology & Anthropology and the Institute of Criminology at the Hebrew University of Jerusalem, "PRRs," or "proportional reporting ratios," are the "lynchpin" of the CDC's VAERS monitoring system.[125] This method compares the proportions of various types of adverse events reported for a new vaccine to those reported for an older, established vaccine. A safety signal is triggered if the reporting rate associated with a new vaccine is much higher for certain adverse events compared to the older one. A safety signal would then trigger an investigation.

However, an article by Guetzkow published in 2022[126] reports that the CDC's response to a FOIA request about its monitoring of VAERS contained a serious admission: "no PRRs were conducted by CDC. Furthermore, data mining is outside of the agency's purview." *How can that be when its own Standard Operating Procedures document cited above says it would "perform PRR data mining on a weekly basis or as needed"?* Gueztkow also noted that CDC officials had repeatedly claimed they had not seen any safety signals in VAERS. The above response by the CDC appears to explain why – *they were not even looking!* When Guetzkow did the PRR calculations himself, the safety signals were there. What makes the CDC's failure even more egregious is that, according to Gueztkow, the CDC had automated the PRR calculations years earlier, so all it had to do was press a button. *How many unnecessary deaths and serious injuries resulted because the CDC withheld important safety data and failed to "press a button"?*

In an article dated September 10, 2022, it was reported that the CDC initially denied that it had made any such calculations, but later acknowledged that it had, starting in February 2021.[127] However, according to that article, the CDC later admitted that it did not start performing PRRs *until March 2022. What seems to be the CDC's problem here?*

As if that were not bad or confusing enough, the same article also reported that the FDA was refusing to release documents relating to a similar data mining process (for Empirical Bayesian data) that it was supposed to have been performing at least bi-weekly, according to the same Standard Operating Procedures document cited above. With regard to a request made by *The Epoch Times* in July 2022 for documents relating to those calculations, the September 10 article reported that the FDA's response was: **"it would not provide any of the analyses, even in redacted form."** Draw your own conclusions.

In August 2022, it was reported that the CDC is also now "admitting it gave false information about reports of adverse events following COVID vaccine surveillance, including inaccurately saying it conducted a certain type of analysis more than one year before it actually did."[128] The CDC says it is now issuing corrections after revisiting many FOIA requests. While it claims the false information was not intentional, the truth has come too late for many.

Might all of these various problems with the CDC be explained at least in part by the CDC's huge conflicts of interest? In 2017. intellectual property expert Mark Blaxill researched the patent ownership of various vaccines. His research showed that as of that time, **the CDC had an ownership interest in 56 vaccine patents.**[129] The Children's Health Defense organization (CHD) further reports that the CDC "buys and distributes $4.6 billion in vaccines annually through the Vaccines for Children program, which is over 40% of its total budget."[130] The same CHD report also quotes UCLA Professor of Medicine Jerome R. Hoffman as saying: "most of us were shocked to learn the CDC takes funding from industry... It is outrageous that industry is apparently allowed to punish the CDC if the agency conducts research that has potential to cut into profits."

The FDA has similar conflicts of interest. According to the FDA website, in 2021 it received 46% of its budget from "industry user fees."[131] It is further reported in a *JAMA* article that in 2018, the amount collected by the FDA in user fees paid 80% of the review personnel's salaries![132]

V-Safe Safety Monitoring Database

In addition to VAERS, the CDC has also maintained another voluntary COVID vaccine safety database called V-safe. V-safe involves use of a phone app to report a person's conditions after receiving the COVID shots. However, the CDC refused to disclose the data until October 2022 when it was forced to do so by a court.[133] The Informed Consent Action Network (ICAN), represented by attorney Aaron Siri, had been trying through multiple legal demands for 15 months to obtain that data. According to one report, ICAN "had to file two lawsuits and multiple appeals to get the CDC to hand it over, and when you see the data, you understand why."[134] Siri states that the CDC could have provided the data in just minutes at any point. ICAN has provided an online searchable database of the V-safe data.[135] Some of the data, based on a total of 10 million participants, are:

- 33.1% (3.31 million) suffered a significant adverse event
- 7.7% (770,000) required medical care after getting the shot
- 25% (2.5 million people) missed work or school or suffered a serious side effect that affected their day-to-day life.
- 40% (or 4 million) reported joint pain (2 million reported it as "moderate" and 400,000 reported it as "severe")"

The CDC reportedly stopped promoting the use of V-safe around May of 2021. *Why might they do that? Why did the CDC withhold and fight not to disclose this important safety information to the public for 15 months?* Let the data speak for themselves.

VAERS Reporting Requirements and Compliance

The law requires reporting of all "serious adverse events" (SAEs) to VAERS by all healthcare providers who administer COVID-19 vaccines, and those who become aware of such events, "regardless of whether the reporter thinks the vaccine caused the AE."[136] "Serious adverse events" as defined by the FDA include death, life-threatening AEs, hospitalization or prolongation of existing hospitalization, persistent or significant incapacity or substantial disruption of the ability to conduct normal life functions, congenital anomalies/birth defects and certain other problems. Healthcare providers are also "encouraged" to report "any additionally clinically significant AEs following vaccination, even if they are not sure whether the vaccine caused the event."

Despite the legal reporting requirement, many health care workers have said that no one in their hospitals has been reporting adverse events following COVID vaccines.[137] Some have said that staff are not told they need to, or are not trained how to make a report. *Might many have been too intimidated by their superiors and too fearful of what might happen to them if they submitted a report? Why would top hospital staff discourage their personnel from submitting a report required by federal law? Should they not be encouraging compliance in order to provide more accurate safety data that would benefit everyone?*

Perhaps the problem is explained by the testimony of a military physician-whistleblower, LTC Theresa M. Long, MD, MPH, FS, under oath in the Seals 1 v. Austin court case, when she kept answering questions posed by lead counsel by saying that she had been ordered not to answer, including with respect to military medical data. When Judge Merryday demanded to know who was ordering her not to testify, she disclosed that she was "ordered by her command" not to testify about any military data. She also testified that she feared for the life and safety of her family and children.[138]

If you have your "juror" hat on, do you think an intelligent person like this doctor would dare make such a statement under oath in court if it were not true? Think of all the huge risks to her own career and her family she was taking. *Based on LTC Long's testimony, what are we to make of any statement coming from the Biden administration concerning the safety and effectiveness of these shots?*

Despite the risk of imprisonment, LTC Long did go on to testify as directed by Judge Merryday. She attributed her courage to testify to praying the night before the trial and waking up at 3:00 a.m. with the Scripture from Leviticus 5:1 on her heart. Leviticus 5:1 states: "If you are called to testify about something you have seen or that you know about, it is sinful to refuse to testify, and you will be punished for your sin."[139] That is just one of many ways God speaks to us, to encourage and embolden us.

[123] https://www.cdc.gov/coronavirus/2019-ncov/vaccines/safety/adverse-events.html (last accessed Aug. 12, 2022)

[124] https://www.cdc.gov/vaccinesafety/pdf/VAERS-v2-SOP.pdf, section 2.3.1 (Jan. 29, 2021)

[125] Josh Guetzkow, Ph.D., https://childrenshealthdefense.org/defender/cdc-vaers-covid-vaccine-safety (June 6, 2022)

[126] Id.

[127] Zachary Stieber, https://www.theepochtimes.com/exclusive-fda-refuses-to-provide-key-covid-19-vaccine-safety-analyses_4722586.html (Sept. 10, 2022)

[128] Zachary Stieber, https://www.theepochtimes.com/exclusive-cdc-admits-it-gave-false-information-about-covid-19-vaccine-surveillance_4657836.html (Aug. 11, 2022)

[129] Ginger Taylor, https://greenmedinfo.com/blog/examining-rfk-jrs-claim-cdc-owns-over-20-vaccine-patents (Jan. 17, 2017)

[130] https://childrenshealthdefense.org/cdc-who/

[131] https://www.fda.gov/about-fda/fda-basics/fact-sheet-fda-glance (last accessed Sept. 13, 2022)

[132] Darrow JJ, Avorn J, Kesselheim AS. FDA Approval and Regulation of Pharmaceuticals, 1983-2018. *JAMA*. 2020;323(2):164–176. doi:10.1001/jama.2019.20288 1; https://pubmed.ncbi.nlm.nih.gov/31935033/

[133] Dr. Joseph Mercola, https://childrenshealthdefense.org/defender/v-safe-data-cdc-covid-vaccines-dangerous-cola/ (Oct. 18, 2022)

[134] Id.

[135] https://icandecide.org/article/v-safe/

[136] https://www.cdc.gov/vaccinesafety/ensuringsafety/monitoring/vaers/reportingaes.html

[137] Steve Kirsch interview with nurse, https://rumble.com/vtge32-tawny-buettner-rn-observed-a-10x-increase-in-the-rate-of-myocarditis-after-.html (Jan. 28, 2022)

[138] https://ac.news/military-doctor-testifies-she-was-ordered-to-cover-up-vaccine-injuries/(March 31, 2022); https://en-volve.com/2022/03/30/military-doctor-testifies-under-oath-that-she-was-ordered-to-cover-up-vaccine-injuries-through-biden-admin-directive/ (March 30, 2022)

[139] Comments of LTC Theresa Long at the Eagle Forum of California Annual Conference, Foundations of Freedom – God, Family and Country (April 8, 2022)

Chapter 9
VAERS: The Under-Reporting Factor & Causality

It is well-known that adverse events are ***grossly under-reported.*** According to Steve Kirsch, medical philanthropist, COVID researcher and founder of the Vaccine Safety Research Foundation (VSRF), the CDC (as well as the FDA and other government officials) either cannot or will not reveal what they believe is a reasonable under-reporting factor (URF) for vaccines (at least not as of October 2021).[140]

However, the URF has been estimated by several independent researchers and statisticians to vary from a factor of about 10 or 20 (very conservatively) up to 100 or more to 1.[141] The oft-cited Harvard study done in 2010 concluded that "fewer than 1% of vaccine adverse events are reported" to VAERS.[142] That would translate into a URF of ***100x*** the numbers showing in VAERS. An analysis done by VSRF founder Steve Kirsch and his team in 2021 concluded that a reasonable URF estimate for serious AEs was 41.[143] This figure was arrived at in nine different ways, and the article in the last footnote explains how that URF was calculated. However, depending on various factors, that estimate could increase. In fact, in May 2022, Kirsch stated that "the URF [of 41] was calculated for the 'very best case' event, so any practical URF should be higher than 41."[144]

Dr. Jessica Rose, Ph.D., a Canadian researcher with a Bachelor's Degree in Applied Mathematics, a Master's in Immunology, a Ph.D. in Computational Biology and two Post-Doctoral degrees, one in Molecular Biology and one in Biochemistry,[145] estimated in January 2022 that a reasonable URF for VAERS reports of spontaneous abortions is 118.[146] (See her article for her calculation method.)

Kirsch has been accused of being a "superspreader" of COVID misinformation. But ***is*** he? Do you know Steve's story? *[147]* He is a former, highly successful Silicon Valley tech entrepreneur and an engineer with two degrees from MIT. He was double-vaxxed by March 2021. Shortly after, he started hearing stories from friends about their relatives who had suffered permanent disabilities or even died after getting the shots. This prompted him to investigate. The more he looked into it, the more appalled he was by what he saw. He then began an aggressive pursuit of the truth about the COVID shots. He has been devoting himself to researching COVID issues since about mid-2021 and founded the Vaccine Safety Research Foundation. He does many data analyses, as well as interviews of vaccine injury victims, physicians and other experts relating to COVID vaccine safety issues. Kirsch also has repeatedly challenged others to come forward to debate him or to disprove his calculations if they are so sure he is spreading misinformation. There have been no takers so far.

Albert Benavides is perhaps the most knowledgeable VAERS expert in the world, with over 26 years of experience as a professional systems data analyst and auditor. He believes that a more accurate URF for VAERS (as of August 2022), is much higher than 41.[148] This is because of new data since Kirsch did his original calculations, such as the reports from life insurance companies and increases in all-cause mortality, as well as other factors. Benavides believes that the early Harvard study (concluding that less than 1% of adverse reactions were reported to VAERS) was probably more correct, and today may even be a conservative estimate. Therefore, he supports the 118 URF for spontaneous abortions cited by Rose above. In fact, he suggests that the current death count in VAERS (as of August 2022) could be doubled and then multiplied by Kirsch's URF of 41 to arrive at a more reasonable estimate.[149]

Despite the differences in the various estimated URFs over the past year or so, whether it is 41 or over 100 does not change how the government, the manufacturers and the major media should have been responding to the warning signals from VAERS that have been blaring since January of 2021.

Some of the other reasons cited by Benavides as to why even a URF of 41 is now much too low include the following: 1) there has been an excessive lag time in the publication of the data by VAERS – several months, even up to a year, even though the VAERS website says it takes about 4-6 weeks to publish; and 2) the fact that since 2011, VAERS only publishes the *initial* reports regarding a particular person, not any updated reports.[150] That means, for example, if an initial VAERS report showed only a serious injury, but the person later died from the injury, that death would *not* show up in the published VAERS death numbers, even if an updated reported had been filed. According to Benavides, the CDC and the FDA continue to collect follow up data, but they do not publish it. He says that this "introduces a new paradigm into the Under-Reporting Factor (URF) by asking a simple question: *how many people who initially reported only a non-death injury to VAERS have since died?*"[151] The answer is, of course, no one knows.

Given the huge number of initial reports of adverse events, **857,343 as of August 12, 2022 just for the U.S. alone,**[152] **and only 14,061 reported U.S. deaths as of that dat**e, it is highly likely that a significant number of the AEs later had a death outcome. The published figure for U.S. deaths alone is *less than half* of the *total* deaths published in VAERS, and the number of AE reports for the U.S. represents only about 60% of the total in VAERS.[153]

Benavides also provided other evidence that suggests VAERS is being purposely "throttled" by the FDA and CDC. He described it as various kinds of data manipulation, including deletion of deaths and other severe adverse event reports, "bundling" of deaths into single cases, and hiding vital pieces of data in the reports that make searches much more difficult, among many other tactics.

Causality

A VAERS report *alone* may not be enough to *prove* causality, but some factors even by themselves are highly indicative of causation. When taken together, they reveal very compelling evidence of causation. Steve Kirsch has stated: "Those who believe the FDA mantra that you cannot use VAERS to determine causality, should start by reading this editorial: 'If Vaccine Adverse Events Tracking Systems Do Not Support Causal Inference, then 'Pharmacovigilance' Does Not Exist.'"[154]

One key takeaway from the editorial Kirsch cites is the amount of time it takes for vaccine-injury victims to get a ruling on causality in the U.S. National Vaccine Injury Compensation Program.[155] In some cases, the author James Lyons-Weiler, PhD, notes, the debates between the experts go on for over 10 years! He then contrasts that with how quickly it was determined that adverse events in the clinical trials were not connected to the vaccine. Since the rollout, that is still the case with many physicians. ***How have they determined so quickly that their patients' conditions are NOT vaccine-related?***

Dr. Peter McCullough has considered all of the Bradford-Hill tenets of causality and concluded: "It is beyond any shadow of a doubt that the vaccines are causing large numbers of deaths." [156] Moreover, as a cardiologist, he has also asserted:

> "We're seeing sudden death now on a massive scale in younger people. . . . If a healthy person dies and there's no antecedent disease, it's the vaccine until proven otherwise."[157]

That is a conservative approach, he said, because the majority of American adults have received the COVID shots. The same sentiment has been expressed by cardiologist Dr. Aseem Malhotra, who said: "Until proven otherwise, it is likely that Covid mRNA vaccines played a significant or primary role in all unexplained heart attacks, strokes, cardiac arrhythmias and heart failure since 2021." [158] The Vaccine Safety Research Foundation has released a powerful 4-minute video on this topic entitled "Until Proven Otherwise."[159]

A close time proximity of a reaction to the time of injection makes causality much more likely. In addition, the person reporting the event must have had a good reason to believe it was vaccine-related. Otherwise, why bother? Knowingly filing a false report is punishable by huge fines and possible imprisonment. According to McCullough, 60-80% of VAERS reports are submitted by health care providers (which can be verified by reading the reports)[160] and that reflects a fairly high likelihood of causation in the reports actually submitted.

The sheer numbers of adverse events all occurring so soon after vaccination is also strong evidence of a causal link. The fact that Pfizer had to hire at least 1,800 more full-time employees just to handle AE reports starting in the 1st quarter 2021very shortly after the vaccine rollout is more strong evidence of causation.[161] In addition, a study done in 2021 found that in only 14% of the deaths reported to VAERS following COVID vaccinations could the vaccine be ruled out as a causal factor in the reports studied. That means that it likely was a causal factor in 86% of the deaths studied.[162]

---

[140] Steve Kirsch, https://www.trialsitenews.com/a/why-wont-the-cdc-or-fda-reveal-the-vaers-urf (Oct. 25, 2021)

[141] See, e.g., Ronald N. Kostoff, PhD, et al, "Why are We Vaccinating Children Against COVID-19?" https://www.sciencedirect.com/science/article/pii/S221475002100161X#bib002 (2021)

[142] https://openvaers.com/images/r18hs017045-lazarus-final-report-20116.pdf (2010)

[143] Steve Kirsch, Jessica Rose and Matthew Crawford https://www.skirsch.com/covid/Deaths.pdf (updated Dec. 24, 2021)

[144] https://stevekirsch.substack.com/p/jackpot-over-500000-killed-by-the?utm_source=email&s=r (May 13, 2022)

[145] https://www.voiceforscienceandsolidarity.org/authors/jessica-rose

[146] https://jessicar.substack.com/p/the-true-under-reporting-factor-urf (1/28/22)

[147] https://stevekirsch.substack.com/about

[148] Albert Benavides interviewed by Dr. James A. Thorp, Aug. 4, 2022.

[149] Personal correspondence between Albert Benavides and Dr. James Thorp, Aug. 2022

[150] Id.

[151] Personal correspondence between Albert Benavides & Dr. James Thorp (11/2/22)

[152] https://openvaers.com/covid-data as of Aug.12, 2022

[153] Id.

[154] https://www.skirsch.com/covid/Deaths.pdf (last update: Dec. 24, 2021), p. 3

[155] James Lyons-Weiler, Ph.D., Editorial: "If Vaccine Adverse Events Tracking Systems Do Not Support Causal Inference, then "Pharmacovigilance" Does Not Exist," *Science Public Health Policy and the Law*, Volume 3:81–86, https://cf5e727d-d02d-4d71-89ff-9fe2d3ad957f.filesusr.com/ugd/adf864_4588b37931024c5d98e35a84acf8069a.pdf (Aug. 2021), pp. 82-83

[156] https://sage.gab.com/channel/constitution1a/view/dr-peter-mccullough-im-telling-624c83ef7fc2d0efc8a3eb2d (2/3/22)

[157] https://rumble.com/embed/v1kydtw/?pub=4

[158] Will Jones, https://www.sott.net/article/473313-Until-proven-otherwise-it-is-likely-Covid-mRNA-vaccines-played-a-significant-role-in-all-unexplained-heart-attacks-since-2021-renowned-cardiologist (Oct. 18, 2022)

[159] https://twitter.com/DrAseemMalhotra/status/1588396524362665987?s=20&utm_source=substack&utm_medium=email

[160] Steve Kirsch, https://stevekirsch.substack.com/p/the-great-debate-politifact-vs-the (Feb. 25, 2022)

[161] EthanH, "Latest Pfizer document dump shows the company had to hire 2,400 more employees to handle wave of COVID "vaccine" adverse events, https://citizens.news/607699.html (April 6, 2022)..

[162] McLachlan, Scott; Osman, Magda, et al, "Analysis of COVID-19 vaccine death reports from the Vaccine Adverse Events Reporting System (VAERS) Database Interim: Results and Analysis," https://www.researchgate.net/publication/352837543; DOI:10.13140/RG.2.2.26987.26402 (June 2021)

Chapter 10
VAERS Data Comparisons

Since adverse events have *always* been under-reported, the VAERS data are still valid for purposes of comparisons, trends and warnings. These data still offer an "apples to apples" comparison. The main problem with VAERS data is in trying to determine ***actual*** numbers or ***more accurate estimates*** of AEs because of the vast under-reporting and the various forms of data manipulation by the government.

Comparisons with Previous Vaccine Reports

Consider the CDC's VAERS data presented in the opening pages of Part 1 (same as Table 7 below) comparing even just ONE year of COVID data with that of ALL other vaccines COMBINED over the previous 30 YEARS, and then the updated data in Table 8 below.

Table 7. VAERS data (for only the U.S.): Comparing adverse event (AE) reports following COVID-19 shots for the first 12 months with the COMBINED TOTAL of AEs reported for ALL other vaccines over the 30 yr. period prior to COVID vaccine rollout[163] (NOTE: no *under-reporting* factor has been applied)

VAERS DATA as of Dec 31, 2021 (For the U.S. only)	30 yrs 1990-2020 for all other vaccinations COMBINED (U.S. only)	COVID-19 vaccines in 1 year (U.S. only)
Adverse reactions	754,900	715,857
Life threatening events	9,903	11,066
Hospitalizations	38,790	46,755
Deaths	5,241	9,778
Permanent disabilities	12,804	11,413

Table 8 below reveals the degree of changes between *average monthly* COVID-19 vaccine VAERS numbers from rollout through the end of 2021 and the average monthly numbers for the first 7 months of 2022, through July

29.[164] Notice the huge decrease in the monthly averages of every category of serious AEs between the 2021 and the 2022 data.

Table 8. Comparison of monthly averages of VAERS reports following COVID-19 vaccines (*for the U.S. only*) from rollout in mid-December, 2020 through Dec. 31, 2021 (12.5 mos.) and January 1 through July 29, 2022.

VAERS reports by category (for U.S. only)	Col. 1 COVID-19 Vax thru 12/31/2021	Col. 2 COVID-19 Vax from rollout thru 7/29/2022	Total reported in 2022 only (Col. 2 minus Col.1)	Monthly ave. from rollout thru 12/31/2021 (12.5 mos.)	Monthly ave. 1/1/2022 to 7/29/2022 (7 mos.)
Adverse reactions	715,857	851,369	135,512	57,269	19,359
Life threatening events	11,066	12,954	1,888	885	270
Hospitalizations	46,755	66,332	19,577	3,740	2,797
Deaths	9,778	13,894	4,116	782	588
Permanent disabilities	11,413	14,536	3,123	913	446

Keep in mind that the above numbers are raw data. There has been no under-reporting factor applied. While some may suggest that the large decreases in the monthly average show that the vaccines were proving to be either more effective or less dangerous (or both) in 2022, the rest of the data and other information in this Part 2 do not support that suggestion. Rather, these significant decreases suggest serious irregularities in VAERS, including an excessive lag time in publication by VAERS, and factors resulting in even significantly fewer reports of deaths and other AEs being submitted to or being published by VAERS. The latter would mean that the appropriate under-reporting factor should be higher.

Do you consider it "misinformation" for Dr. Peter McCullough to conclude on the basis of that data that the COVID vaccines are "the most dangerous biological medicinal product rollout in human history?" Given that those data show that the number of deaths reported in only 1 year for COVID vaccines was *almost 2X* the total number of deaths following ALL other vaccines COMBINED over the previous 30 years, *is that "misinformation?"* What about the other data, shown in Table 3 of Part 1, comparing the *average annual* number of adverse events and deaths reported in VAERS *over the last 10 years* with 1 year of COVID data showing increases of 1,800% and 6,000%, respectively? *How is it "misinformation" if a person is simply reporting the government's own data and then making an obvious comparison?*

Total Number of American Deaths and Other AEs After COVID Shots

See the following Table 9 applying the Kirsch team's now rather low URF of 41, and Benavides' suggested URF of 100, based on the reported VAERS updated adverse event and death counts for the U.S. alone as of September 12, 2022.[165] The CDC continues to claim that "reports of death after COVID-19 vaccination *are rare."* [166] What seems relatively "rare" is how many are actually reported and published in VAERS. *How do you explain such a huge discrepancy?*

Table 9. Estimated actual number of Deaths and other Adverse Events for the U.S. only through Sept. 12, 2022 using URFs applied to VAERS data

VAERS: U.S.-only data after COVID shots	Totals from rollout in Dec. 2020 thru Sept. 12, 2022	Applying a URF of 41	Applying a URF of 100
Adverse events	867,527	Many millions	Many millions
Deaths	14,528	**595,648**	**1,452,800**

1976 Swine Flu Vaccine Comparison

You may remember the 1976 swine flu crisis. The government initiated a vaccination campaign in October that year, but the campaign was ended shortly thereafter in December 1976 due to the number of adverse events. That number was massively less than the number of AEs from COVID-19. Dr Peter McCullough has reported that the number of deaths at the time the campaign was ended was only 25.[167] The *60 Minutes* program had a whole episode about this in late 1979.[168] In 1976, the government had warned that swine flu could turn into a killer outbreak nationwide. They encouraged every adult and child to get a vaccine to prevent a pandemic.

Sound familiar? More than 40 million did so. The moderator reported that by far the greatest number of claims from these swine flu shots were for neurological damage, or even death. A very important admission about this on the CDC website[169] includes the following statement as to why that vaccine was stopped after only a couple months:

> "In 1976 there was a ***small increased risk*** of a serious neurological disorder called Guillain-Barré Syndrome (GBS) following vaccination with a swine flu vaccine. The increased risk was approximately 1 additional case of GBS for every 100,000 people who got the swine flu vaccine. When over 40 million people were vaccinated against swine flu, federal health officials decided that ***the possibility of an association of GBS with the vaccine, however small, necessitated stopping immunization until the issue could be explored.***" *(*emphasis added)

In that vaccination campaign, just the "possibility, however small" of an association with a disease as serious as GBS "necessitated stopping immunization until the issue could be explored." The numbers of reported adverse reactions, deaths and serious injuries are exponentially higher with the COVID shots. ***Why is it that in 1976 only a "small number" of GBS cases was enough to stop the vaccine campaign, but as of the summer of 2022, when more than 800,000 adverse events and more than 14,000 deaths had been reported to VAERS in the U.S. alone,[170] the government is not only still encouraging the shots, but even mandating them for various groups?***

Here we are, almost two years later, with countless more deaths and serious injuries than in 1976, and government officials are doing NOTHING even to pause, much less to stop the vaccine campaign. The fact that the FDA has now authorized these shots for young children as young as 6 months old should seriously concern every parent and grandparent. **See the section below on why doctors all over the world have warned governments** *not to give these shots to children.*

Dr. Peter McCullough has extensive experience with drug review boards, including vaccines. In an interview with renowned podcaster Joe Rogan in December 2021, McCullough stated many important facts. Here is a short summary by Dr. Joseph Mercola of a few of those points: [171]

"Historically, any drug with five unexplained deaths gets a black box warning. At 50 unresolved deaths, it's pulled from the market altogether. None of that happened here. To this day, the FDA and CDC claim not a single death is attributable to the COVID shots, even as the reported death toll is nearing 20,000[12] (including international reports), with half of them occurring within 48 hours of the injection. Eighty percent occur within a week post-injection.

"That is simply unheard of. The temporal association is stronger than anything we've seen before. McCullough also cites research concluding that in 86% of cases, there was no other explanation for the death other than the COVID shot."

Where was the black box warning with these shots? According to the data,[172] a death count of 50 was reached by January 2021, in the month following the rollout. Why was no action taken way back then?

---

[163] https://openvaers.com/covid-data (as of July 29, 2022)

[164] Id.

[165] www.openvaers.com, as of Sept. 12, 2022

[166] https://www.cdc.gov/coronavirus/2019-ncov/vaccines/safety/adverse-events.html

[167] https://thenewamerican.com/covid-shot-killing-large-numbers-warns-top-covid-doc-peter-mccullough/ (April 27, 2021)

[168] https://childrenshealthdefense.org/video/60-minutes-swine-flu-1976-vaccine-warning/ (Aired on *60 Minutes* on Nov. 4, 1979)

[169] https://www.cdc.gov/vaccinesafety/concerns/concerns-history.html

[170] https://openvaers.com/covid-data (as of June 24, 2022)

[171] Dr. Joseph Mercola, notes of Dr. Peter McCullough's interview by Joe Rogan, "The Most Important Podcast You Can Hear About COVID-19," https://takecontrol.substack.com/p/understanding-covid-19?s=r (Dec. 23, 2021)

[172] https://openvaers.com/covid-data/mortality

Chapter 11

Early Pfizer Documents:
The "75-Year Delay" & the First 3-Month Report

The FDA's Attempt to Delay up to 75 Years to Release Pfizer Documents

Four days after the Pfizer/Comirnaty vaccine was reported to have been "fully approved" by the FDA in August of 2021, a group of health care professionals made a Freedom of Information Act request to the FDA. It sought documents the FDA relied on in making that decision.[173]

The group requested expedited processing based on the urgency of the matter for those who were facing vaccine mandates. *The FDA refused the expedited processing on the ground that there was "no compelling need that involves an imminent threat to the life or safety of an individual."*[174] Ask any of the countless injured health care personnel, military members, pilots and others subjected to the mandates if they agree with that.

The FDA proposed a timeline to release 500 documents per month. At that rate, given the estimated total pages, it would have taken 75 years to produce all of the documents! Fortunately, the court gave the FDA only eight months. The Plaintiff's attorney, Aaron Siri, said that the FDA's position is even more inexcusable because:

> "The FDA licensed the Pfizer vaccine ... just 108 days after Pfizer started producing the records to the agency. During that period, the FDA asserts it conducted an intense, robust, and thorough analysis ... to assure the public that the Pfizer vaccine was safe and effective. Yet, when asked to share those documents with the public, the FDA claimed it needed over 20,000 days."[175]

In addition, the attorney noted that the FDA has over 18,000 employees and a budget of $6.5 billion, yet it tried to tell the judge that it had limited resources to produce the documents any faster. *If the vaccines are as safe and effective as they claim, why would the FDA seek to drag out the release of documents for up to 75 years? Should they not be eager to prove the basis for that claim sooner rather than later?*

The monumental task of reviewing the hundreds of thousands of pages has been done under the leadership of Naomi Wolf, author of *The Bodies of Others: The New Authoritarians, COVID-19 and the War Against the Human,* released in 2022. Generally, according to Wolf, the documents show "massive general harm" during the clinical trials, especially regarding reproduction.[176] The documents can be viewed at her company's website, www.DailyClout.com.[177]

Pfizer Data Showing Adverse Events Through 2/28/21

One of the earliest documents released by the FDA about its review of Pfizer documents was entitled "5.3.6 Cumulative Analysis of Post-Authorization Adverse Event Reports of PF-07302048 (BNT162B2) Received Through 28-Feb-2021."[178] It covered the first 90 days after the vaccine rollout. The report was delivered to the federal government on April 30, 2021, so they had at least "constructive knowledge" of its contents by that date. However, it was not made available to the public until late in 2021, about seven months after the government received it.

Dr. Jessica Rose, Ph.D., the highly-credentialed Canadian scientist and researcher cited above, reviewed this document. She pointed out that the number of adverse events reported to VAERS for this time frame (regarding the Pfizer products) was 84,770, *"literally twice the N [number] reported by Pfizer in their report."*[179] Putting that big discrepancy aside and using the numbers in the Pfizer report, the data should still have sent signals concerning safety based on what was known in the first 3 months.

Dr. Daniel Nagase, a Canadian emergency room doctor, explained some highlights of that document.[180] Table 10 below shows the breakdown of the recovery status of the 42,086 adverse events reported in the first few months after the rollout. Note that the total of the three categories of people who had not fully recovered represent nearly 31% of the total number of AEs. Potentially a significant number of the cases where the recovery status was unknown may also have been unresolved. That would increase the percentage of unresolved cases even more. ***These data were known by Pfizer and the government in early 2021, yet there was no response by either.***

Table 10: Select Data from Pfizer's *5.3.6 Cumulative Analysis of Post-Authorization Adverse Event Reports of PF-07302048 (BNT162B2) Received Through 28-Feb-2021 (since the December 2020 rollout)* [181]

Total # of adverse events 1st 3 mos.	Col. A Not recovered	Col. B Recovered with Sequelae	Col. C Deaths	Total of Col. A, B & C	Recovery status "unknown"
42,806	11,361	520	1,223	13,104	9,400

Appendix 1 in that 30-page Pfizer "5.3.6 Cumulative Analysis" has almost 9 full pages listing nearly 1,300 kinds of "special interest adverse events" identified with their vaccine in the first *three months*. This was one of the documents Pfizer used to get its Comirnaty product license application approved by the FDA in August, 2021, despite the adverse event data just presented. Yet page 28 of the report says that "Pfizer performs frequent and rigorous signal detection on BNT162b2 [COVID vaccine] cases," and their conclusion was:

> "The data do not reveal any novel safety concerns or risks requiring label changes and support a favorable benefit risk profile of to the BNT162b2 vaccine. Review of the available data for this cumulative PM experience, confirms a favorable benefit: risk balance for BNT162b2."

It makes one wonder who was reviewing this data, what standards they were applying and what their motives were to ignore blaring safety signals!

---

[173] https://phmpt.org/wp-content/uploads/2021/11/091621-Complaint.pdf
[174] Ibid, p. 3
[175] Edward Hendrie, https://greatmountainpublishing.com/2021/11/23/the-fda-took-108-days-to-review-pfizer-documents-before-approving-its-covid-19-vaccine-but-the-fda-wants-to-take-55-years-to-review-those-same-documents-before-releasing-them-to-the-public/ (Nov. 23, 2021)
[176] Art Moore, https://www.wnd.com/2022/10/naomi-wolf-elites-covering-deadly-vax-complicit-massive-crime/ Oct.1, 2022)
[177] https://campaigns.dailyclout.io/campaign/brand/cc3b3e5a-6536-4738-8ed6-5ee368c67240
[178] https://phmpt.org/wp-content/uploads/2021/11/5.3.6-postmarketing-experience.pdf
[179] https://jessicar.substack.com/p/pfizer-adverse-event-data (Dec. 5, 2021)
[180] Dr. Daniel Nagase interviewed on Strong and Free Truthcast https://rumble.com/vqq3hw-breaking-news-pfizers-own-stats-1200-40000-trial-participants-dead-intervie.html (Dec. 13, 2021)
[181] https://phmpt.org/wp-content/uploads/2021/11/5.3.6-postmarketing-experience.pdf, p. 7

Chapter 12
Adverse Impacts on Pregnancy & Breastfeeding

According to one of this book's contributing authors, Ob-Gyn and maternal-fetal specialist Dr. James A. Thorp, giving the COVID shots to pregnant women is an egregious violation of the "golden rule" of pregnancy. That rule is: *experimental drugs and new substances should never, ever be given to a pregnant or lactating woman.* Thorp explains the basis for this rule:

> "It is now widely known and understood that the COVID-19 "vaccine," which is an experimental gene therapy, works by inducing inflammation. Yet, inflammation in the developing embryo and fetus is a hallmark for permanent damage, malformation, death, placental insufficiency, and potentially life long chronic diseases in the offspring, including severe immunological disturbances, disruption of the TOL7 and TOL8 receptors on cell membranes." [182]

Thorp has also stated that the recommendation of this vaccine for pregnant women by the American Board of Obstetrics and Gynecology "may well be the greatest disaster in the history of obstetrics."[183] In contrast, at least as of August 2022, the UK government issued a Summary of the Public Assessment Report for the Pfizer vaccine in the UK which specifically states that "sufficient reassurance of safe use of the vaccine in pregnant women *cannot be provided at the present time"* and also that *"women who are breastfeeding should not be vaccinated."*[184] However, other UK government website pages offer contrary advice, stating: "COVID-19 vaccination is strongly recommended for pregnant and breastfeeding women."[185]

Pregnancy Outcome Data From the Pfizer Report Ending 2/28/21

Dr. Thorp, Dr. Nagase and Dr. Rose, as well as many others, were quite alarmed at what was revealed in the "Missing Information" section of Pfizer's "5.3.6 Cumulative Analysis" document (cited above) about pregnancy outcomes of women who were vaccinated during the first three months of the rollout. The data on page 12 of that report show there were 270 pregnancies, but "no outcome was provided for 238" of them, for reasons which the report does not explain.[186] *What happened to those 238?*

For the remaining 32, about which some pregnancy outcome information was provided, the data were presented in a very sloppy and confusing way. In addition, the report includes more than one set of different descriptions and inconsistent numbers of various adverse events that do not add up, and of those 32, the outcome was listed as "pending" for 5 of them. Moreover, according to Ob-Gyn specialist Dr. James A. Thorp, the terms that obstetrical clinicians use are poorly understood by other physicians and health care providers, as well as by those who submit reports to VAERS and write the Pfizer documents. Nevertheless, the best that Thorp is able to discern from the Pfizer report writer's struggle with appropriate terminology are the following:

124 of 270 pregnant women reported "adverse events" (46%)
75 of those 270 women reported "serious adverse events" (27%)

Pregnancy Outcomes: (among the 32 for whom some information was provided)

- 1 "normal outcome" (1/32 or 3%)
- 1 "foetal death" (1/32 = 3%)
- 25 miscarriages ("abortion spontaneous")(25/32 = **78% miscarriage rate**)

TOTAL deaths: 25 miscarriages + 1 foetal death = 26/32 = **81%**

According to the CDC, a typical miscarriage rate is about 11-16%.[187] Therefore, regardless of what the outcomes of the 5 pending pregnancies were, the deaths so greatly outnumber the "normal outcomes" that there is no rational basis upon which anyone could conclude that these shots are safe for pregnant women. Nonetheless, despite the alarming rates of miscarriage and total death outcomes and *only 1 known normal outcome,* Pfizer's conclusion to this summary of "Missing Information" was: *"There were no safety signals that emerged from the review of these cases of use in pregnancy…."*[188] The FDA and CDC totally ignored the blaring safety signals and allowed Pfizer to get away with a blatantly dishonest conclusion.

More Recent Pregnancy Data. In a study intended to evaluate vaccine safety during pregnancy, Shimabukuro et al followed outcomes in 3,958 vaccinated pregnant women between mid-December 2020 and the end of

February 2021.[189] During the two-and-a-half-month period, 827 women completed their pregnancy of which 712 (86.1%) were live births and 115 (13.9%) were pregnancy losses. Of the pregnancy losses, 104 were spontaneous abortions, the vast majority of which (92.3%) occurred before 13 weeks of gestation. Upon review of the data, however, 700 (84.6%) of women were not vaccinated until the third trimester, and therefore should not have been included in the calculation of spontaneous abortions. That is because spontaneous abortions (or miscarriages), by definition, only include deaths of the baby during the first 20 weeks.

Based on their misleading calculations, they pegged the spontaneous abortion rate at 12.6% (104/827), right in line with the CDC's typical range of 11-16%,[190] when, in fact, it was actually 82% (104/127). According to Dr. James Thorp, this astonishing miscarriage rate is equivalent to the efficacy of the so-called abortion pill, RU486, which carries an FDA black box warning to alert consumers to major drug risks. And yet Shimabukuro et al concluded there were no obvious safety concerns.

Thorp also characterizes these results as disinformation, plain and simple, and cannot be written off as an accident. He noted that there were 21 named authors on the study, 8 of whom were physicians, including three Ob-Gyn specialists, and others with expertise in public health and epidemiology. It is inconceivable, he suggests, that an error of this magnitude could escape the scrutiny of such a stellar cast. *How could it have been overlooked by the NEJM editorial staff and reviewers unless by intention?* Provocatively, he notes, all 21 authors report affiliations with either CDC or the FDA. And *NEJM*, the flagship journal of the medical-industrial complex, has taken a strong pro-vax stance that can hardly be called objective. Thorp states that Shimabukuro's thinly-veiled attempt to downplay the risks of COVID-19 vaccines and mitigate vaccine hesitancy is yet another research scandal laden with conflicts of interest and intent to deceive. He also suggests that this paper by Shimabukuro et al is "eerily similar" to the ***Pfizer*** "5.3.6 Cumulative Analysis" report discussed above, causing him to wonder if Pfizer may have had a hand in "ghost-writing" this *NEJM* article.

Thorp, Price and Deskevich, et al performed a retrospective cohort study by using VAERS database from January 1, 1998 to June 30, 2022. It was published September 28, 2022.[191] The obstetrical complications after the COVID-19 vaccines were compared to those after Influenza vaccines. There were substantial increases in menstrual abnormalities, miscarriage, fetal malformations, fetal chromosomal abnormalities, fetal cystic hygroma, fetal growth restriction, fetal cardiac abnormalities, fetal cardiac arrhythmia, fetal cardiac arrest, placental thrombosis, fetal growth restriction, fetal vascular mal-perfusion, oligohydramnios, abnormalities of fetal surveillance and fetal deaths. All of these abnormalities were clinically and statistically significant and, in fact, were corroborated by multiple completely independent sources worldwide.

Table 11 below,[192] also reported in Part 1, compares pregnancy losses reported to VAERS following COVID shots over 20 months vs. flu shots over 32.5 years. This evidence flies in the face of Shimabukuro's claim that the vaccines are safe during pregnancy.

Table 11. Nearly 168 X the annual average # of pregnancy losses were reported to VAERS following COVID-19 vaccines in 20 months than reported after flu shots in the past 32.5 years. (p value < 0.0001) *(the following are the raw data before any under-reporting factor is applied)*

As of Aug, 9, 2022, by type of pregnancy loss	FLU VACCINE Total pregnancy losses since 1990 (over 32.5 years)	COVID-19 VACCINE Total pregnancy losses in 20 months (1.66 yrs)
Miscarriages (spontaneous abortions in 1st 20 wks)	396	3,723
Fetal deaths (after 20 wks.)	90	458
TOTAL pregnancy losses –both types	**486**	**4,181**
Average/yr of miscarriages	12	2,242
Average/yr of fetal deaths	2.77	276
TOTAL ave./yr. for both pregnancy loss types	**15**	**2,518**

Imagine what the real number must be when an under-reporting factor is applied. Applying the URF of 118 suggested by Albert Benavides and Jessica Rose would yield a staggering total of *over 493,000 pregnancy losses in the first 20 months after the COVID vaccine rollout.* Even using Kirsch's much lower "best scenario" conservative URF of 41 would yield a total of 171,400 pregnancy losses following COVID shots. *Is even the lower of these numbers acceptable?*

Dr. Daniel Nagase, the Canadian physician quoted earlier, reports some startling statistics for stillbirths.[193] He stated in late 2021 that a worker in a birthing center in Vancouver reported 13 stillbirths in a 24-hour period. In Waterloo, Ontario, he stated that they used to see only about 5 or 6 stillbirths per year, or about one every two months. In contrast, there were 86 stillbirths between January and July of 2021. The article reporting this information also reported that all 86 women had been vaccinated, but Dr. Nagase has shared with the authors that the vaccination status data came to him from a person who had received it from a nurse.[194]

Additionally, the information on the package insert from the "approved" version of the Pfizer/Comirnaty COVID shot said: "'*Available data on COMIRNATY administered to pregnant women are insufficient to inform vaccine-associated risks in pregnancy.*'(Section 8.1)" It also said data was not available about the effects of the shots on breastfed infants or milk production/excretion.[195]

Thorp also commented on a study published online on September 26, 2022 in the *JAMA Pediatric* edition entitled "Detection of Messenger RNA COVID-19 Vaccines in Human Breast Milk."[196] The study involved only 11 lactating women who had received either the Pfizer or Moderna shots. According to the authors, their data "demonstrate for the first time to our knowledge the biodistribution of COVID-19 vaccine mRNA to mammary cells...." Relatively small trace amounts of mRNA were found sporadically in the breast milk of five of the women within 45 hours after vaccination, but the authors concluded that it was still safe for mothers to breastfeed after a COVID shot. However, they stated that "caution is warranted about breastfeeding children younger than 6 months in the first 48 hours after maternal vaccination until more safety studies are conducted."

Thorp raised concerns about their conclusion, as stated in his comments on the subject published in *The Epoch Times*:[197]

> "Even small quantities of messenger RNA could potentially have significant ramifications on the newborn and could potentially be

amplified by the immune system. This is an extremely poor excuse and they are attempting to minimize the implications of this concerning finding. Coming out with such a study 20 months after they've been pushing the vaccine on pregnant women and breastfeeding mothers is unacceptable and is a major breach of science..."

He also says that these are stunning findings for many reasons. It underscores the abnormal stability of the pseudo-uridinated mRNA allowing it to remain intact and functioning for much longer periods of time than natural mRNA. It is also alarming that the pseudo-uridinated mRNA in the vaccine appears to be transported throughout the body inside of extracellular vesicles (EV). It is also likely that the EV may be transported to every other cell in the body and every other bodily fluid.

Although the authors of that study acknowledge the shortcomings of such a small sampling and recommend further studies, there is another factor to consider. As discussed in later sections, both before and after administration of these shots, there have been great inconsistencies in the amount of mRNA in the vials between batches even from the same manufacturer. Therefore, with a much larger sampling, the results could show a much greater adverse impact, if such discrepancies still exist in current vials.

Despite all of the above, and Pfizer's admission that the data were not sufficient to advise about vaccine risks in pregnancy and breastfeeding, why are pregnant and breastfeeding women being advised that these shots are safe for them?

---

[182] Thorp JA, Renz T, Northrup, C, Lively C, Breggin P, Bartlett R, et al. Patient Betrayal: The Corruption of Healthcare, Informed Consent and the Physician-Patient Relationship. G Med Sci. 2022; 3(1): 046-069. https://www.doi.org/10.46766/thegms.medethics.22021403, p. 8

[183] Id.

[184] https://www.gov.uk/government/publications/regulatory-approval-of-pfizer-biontech-vaccine-for-covid-19/summary-public-assessment-report-for-pfizerbiontech-covid-19-vaccine (updated Aug. 16, 2922)

[185] Norman Fenton, https://www.normanfenton.com/post/breaking-news-uk-government-says-vaccine-not-safe-for-pregnant-or-breastfeeding-women (Aug. 29, 2022)

[186] https://phmpt.org/wp-content/uploads/2021/11/5.3.6-postmarketing-experience.pdf, p. 12

[187] https://www.cdc.gov/media/releases/2021/s0811-vaccine-safe-pregnant.html

[188] https://phmpt.org/wp-content/uploads/2021/11/5.3.6-postmarketing-experience.pdf, p. 13

[189] Shimabukuro TT, Kim SY, Myers TR, Moro PL, Oduyebo T, et al; CDC v-safe COVID-19 Pregnancy Registry Team. Preliminary Findings of mRNA Covid-19 Vaccine Safety in Pregnant Persons. N Engl J Med. 2021 Jun 17;384(24):2273-2282. doi: 10.1056/NEJMoa2104983. Epub 2021 Apr 21. Erratum in: N Engl J Med. 2021 Oct 14;385(16):1536. PMID: 33882218; PMCID: PMC8117969. https://web.archive.org/web/20210630220634/https://pubmed.ncbi.nlm.nih.gov/33882218/

[190] https://www.cdc.gov/media/releases/2021/s0811-vaccine-safe-pregnant.html

[191] Thorp, J.A.; Rogers, C.; Deskevich, M.P.; Tankersley, S.; Benavides, A.; Redshaw, M.D.; McCullough, P.A. COVID-19 Vaccines: The Impact on Pregnancy Outcomes and Menstrual Function. Preprints 2022, 2022090430 (doi: 10.20944/preprints202209.0430.v1). https://www.preprints.org/manuscript/202209.0430/v1

[192] Raw data compiled from VAERS by Dr. James A. Thorp, August 2022.

[193] Alicia Powe, https://www.thegatewaypundit.com/2021/12/video-doctor-warns-stillbirths-rampant-among-fully-vaccinated-mothers-launches-investigation/ (Dec. 11, 2021)

[194] Personal communication from Dr. Daniel Nagase to Sally Saxon, Nov. 2022

[195] Sarah Middleton, https://www.naturalhealth365.com/vaers-reveals-massive-increase-in-fetal-deaths-following-maternal-covid-injection.html (April 19, 2022)

[196] Hanna, N, et al. Detection of Messenger RNA Covid-19 Vaccines in Human Breast Milk. *JAMA Pediatr.* 2022. PMID: 36156636; https://pubmed.ncbi.nlm.nih.gov/36156636/

[197] Enrico Trigoso, https://www.theepochtimes.com/covid-vaccines-contaminate-breastmilk-with-mrna-jama-study_4757809.html (Sept. 27, updated Sept. 28, 2022)

Chapter 13
Devastating Impacts on the Military

Some of the most devastating data come from the military. It appears that the military is being decimated by these shots. Examine the data and other information and draw your own conclusions.

Attorney Todd Callender[198] currently represents several military whistleblowers in connection with the COVID vaccine mandates and other vaccine-related issues. He filed the first lawsuit against the US Department of Defense, the Health and Human Services Department and the FDA in August 2021. That case was <u>Robert v. Austin</u>,[199] which sought to stop the "vaccine" mandates in the DOD. Among other results, the suit has led to the DOD backing off from implementing its proposed involuntary immunizations in which unwilling servicemembers would have been physically restrained against their will and injected with the COVID shots. On November 18, 2022, he argued the case in the 10th Circuit Court of Appeals.

Callender has provided much information to the authors about what these courageous service members have stated in various public documents, such as declarations and affidavits signed under oath, or in various public forums.[200] They speak about what their experience has been in seeking to carry out their duties as health care professionals in the military in light of directives that conflict with the ethics of their profession. Much of what he has shared is rather eye-opening. It should raise serious concerns and questions in the minds of every American as to how the military is being run, and why military leaders are ignoring the data and advice of their own health care professionals in matters that are having devastating adverse impacts on the entire military. The transcript of his comments can be accessed through the link at the end of this chapter.

Data From the Military Database

The following data from the Defense Medical Epidemiology Database (DMED) was provided by four military whistleblowers currently represented by Callender. This database is arguably the most accurate epidemiology database in the country, because the DOD uses a single electronic medical records system for all service members. The DMED allows health care providers to perform queries of ICD codes to look for emerging health trends among active-duty military personnel from 1990 until the present.

As told by Callender, the initial searches and compilation of the data below were done by LTC Theresa M. Long, MD, MPH, FS, an Aerospace and Occupational Medicine Specialist and US Army Flight Surgeon who has served in the US Army since 1991. The problems she and other doctors were seeing in their own patients led her to research emerging trends across the entire DOD using ICD codes that had a pathophysiologic basis for disease or adverse events attributable to the concentration of the spike protein as outlined in Pfizer's Biodistribution Study. (That study is discussed further below in the chapter "Dangers of the Spike Protein.")

For example, Dr. Long was seeing an increase in pituitary brain tumors, and Pfizer's Biodistribution Study clearly showed concentration of the pathogenic spike protein in the pituitary. Her data was independently verified by other whistleblowers: LTC Peter Chambers, D.O., MAJ Sam Sigoloff, D.O., and Public Health Officer 1LT Mark Bashaw. All have made sworn declarations of their findings. They did queries for hundreds of ICD codes from 2016-2021, comparing 2021 to the previous 5-year average for various health conditions.

At a hearing on January 24, 2022 conducted by Senator Ron Johnson, the whistleblowers' DMED data was presented by attorney Tom Renz.[201] That same day Senator Johnson sent a letter to Defense Secretary Lloyd Austin directing him to "preserve all records referring, relating, or reported to the Defense Medical Epidemiology Database (DMED)."[202] At that hearing, Sen. Johnson reported that he was aware that the DMED's data regarding myocarditis "had been doctored already," substantially, since the time the data had been collected several months earlier.[203]

Based on whistleblowers' declarations, Senator Johnson sent another letter February 1, 2022, to Secretary Austin setting forth the whistleblower data found in the DMED database.[204] After noting that diagnoses for ***neurological conditions had increased 10X over the 5-year average, from***

82,000 to 863,000 (a 1,000% increase), Johnson listed the increases over that same 5-year average in several other conditions. See Table 12 below.

Table 12. Percentage of increases over the previous 5-year average (2016-2020) in several diseases among military members a year after the COVID vaccine rollout, as of December 2021, reported by Sen. Ron Johnson in a letter to Defense Secretary Lloyd Austin on February 1, 2022.

Condition or Disease	Percentage of increase
Hypertension	2,181%
Diseases of the nervous system	1,048%
Neurological problems	1,000%
Malignant neoplasms of esophagus	894%
Multiple sclerosis	680%
Malignant neoplasm of digestive organs	624%
Guillain Barré	551%
Breast cancer	487%
Malignant neoplasms of thyroid and other endocrine glands	474%
Female infertility	472%
Pulmonary embolism	468%
Migraines	452%
Ovarian dysfunction	437%
Testicular cancer	369%
Tachycardia	302%

. Other whistleblower data reported by Daniel Horowitz include:[205]

    Myocardial infarction   269% increase
    Bell's palsy   291% increase
    Congenital malformations)   156% increase
    (in children of military personnel)

In the VAERS report form there is a special box to check if the report is being made regarding a service member, which allows people to query and compile VAERS reports on service members. Given the military's use of a single electronic medical records system, these VAERS reports are the most easily verifiable vaccine adverse events reports. According to Todd Callender, to date, the DOD has not notified their health care providers or the general public of the frequency, severity and nature of VAERS reports made on service members.[206]

Despite Senator Johnson's request for the DMED data to be preserved, *PolitiFact* reported on January 28 that the DOD was claiming that the data for the five baseline years was wrong, due to a "glitch in the database," and that it was being taken offline to correct it. The data for *2021,* however, according to a DOD spokesperson, was "up to date."[207] Sen. Johnson sent yet another letter on February 8, 2022 to Secretary Austin, referring back to his earlier letter and warning of January 24, that the database should be preserved.[208] He further expressed concern about the alterations mentioned in the *PolitiFact* article: "Specifically, a DoD spokesperson reportedly told *PolitiFact* that the data in DMED 'was incorrect for the years 2016-2020.'"

In a sworn Declaration, 1LT Mark Bashaw stated that on January 31, 2022, a week after Sen. Johnson's roundtable hearing:

> "I went into DMED, and the data had been changed for 2016-2020. I have excel spreadsheets and live video of running the numbers in DMED, both before and after Senator Johnson's roundtable, which are evidence proving the alteration of the data."[209]

If there had been a glitch in the database for those 5 baseline years, how is it that no one caught such serious errors for several years? The problem with the "glitch" theory, according to Callender, is that the prevalence of problems like pulmonary embolisms, strokes, and neurodegeneration in our young healthy military population (18 to 55-year-olds) would be several times higher than the national average (for 18 to 95-year-olds) for the last 5 years and went unnoticed for 5 years, despite a $42 million surveillance system.[210] Since 1LT Bashaw says they have evidence of what the numbers were before the DOD's alterations, it would be quite interesting to see what might happen with this in a court of law.

In light of the above data, it is rather disturbing to read the following in LTC Long's March 9, 2022 Declaration under oath (p. 6) offered in support of Senator Ron Johnson's investigation (that Declaration can be accessed via the link or QR code at the end of this chapter):

> "the weekly COVID-19 update briefs, were shockingly devoid of information regarding vaccine adverse events in the DOD or

nationwide. ... despite the military publishing some of the first research regarding the risk of myocarditis and pericarditis after COVID vaccination, up-to-date information on emerging trends were not presented."

Other Information

There is much other information publicly shared by the whistleblowers concerning how the military has handled COVID vaccine-related issues that would probably surprise, if not shock, most Americans. Todd Callender describes LTC Long as "the right person in a critical position at a defining moment in history." He added that her assignment as a surgeon at Ft. Rucker "proved to be an epidemiologist's gold mine," as she was tasked with doing a monthly review of the health of about 4,000 young 20 to 30-year-old pilots, aircrew members and soldiers. She observed a noticeable increase in rare and unusual medical problems for this age and population after the COVID vaccines were introduced. Callender quotes a statement by LTC Long:

> "'In fifteen years of taking care of soldiers, I have never seen this litany of debilitating and potentially deadly medical conditions that included strokes or TIAs, pericarditis, myocarditis, erratic heart rates, arrhythmias, rapid onset and progression of various cancers, ... suppression of the immune system, unprovoked blood clots in the splenic and portal vein, avascular necrosis of the hip requiring total hip replacement, liver dysfunction, menstrual irregularities, and miscarriages.'"

LTC Long made many attempts to discuss her findings and grave concerns with her command, but they would not listen to her warnings. On November 4, 2021, prior to the January 24, 2022 hearing mentioned above, she was called to testify before Senator Ron Johnson's subcommittee. She stated that *only 12 active-duty service members at that time had actually died of COVID*, and made the following statement: **"I believe the COVID vaccine is a greater threat to soldiers' health and medical readiness than COVID itself."** In later hearings, she noted that the DOD had testified that only 23 (out of 1.4 million) active-duty members and 93 (out of 2.4 million) members in the total force had died of COVID. ***Do you*** *believe these numbers justify a mandate of a new experimental drug with no long-term safety tests for such a large group?*

She also commented on how the military was pressing forward to separate more than 200,000 servicemembers who had rejected the vaccine, stating that removing them from the military for that reason had the same impact as losing them in battle, noting the military had never lost so many in a few months.

At an Army Senior Preventative Medicine Leadership course, LTC Long dared to question the "logic of risking the health of the entire fighting force on a vaccine they only had two months of safety data on when they had only lost 12 active duty servicemembers to COVID." In what Callender described as "a stunning revelation," a senior medical leader commanded LTC Long to get as many soldiers as possible vaccinated, saying that he needed her to do that in order "to get enough data points to determine *if* the vaccine was safe." *Had not the government assured us all before then that they had already determined it was safe?*

LTC Long also testified on other issues, such as the military leaders' use of threats and coercion to get servicemembers vaccinated, in violation of the Nuremberg Code. Callender also shared how LTC Long had pointed out "the glaring breakdown in risk communication," the failure of leadership to tell servicemembers of the known risks of the shots, and how "whistleblower doctors across the country who dared to raise concerns were demonized, censored, silenced, reprimanded and retaliated against."

At the end of her March 9 Declaration, LTC Long asks several penetrating questions, including: *"Why did the DOD leadership risk the entirety of its fighting force in a grand, dangerous, and deadly experiment in violation of its own laws, policies, procedures, and mandate given that the risk of death among the military population from Covid-19 was a .0038% chance?"* [211] That is a question we should all be asking.

Regarding the other three whistleblowers identified above, Callender commented that LTC Peter Chambers was currently receiving treatment for a serious adverse reaction to the shot, but was boldly speaking out on the issues to make people aware of vaccine injuries within the military. MAJ Sam Sigoloff, "for the crime of doing his job," was suspended and removed from clinical care duties. He was later investigated on "trumped up concerns into his medical practice" and subjected to other unjust treatment. His situation is explained more fully in the transcript of

Callender's comments accessible with other whistleblower documents through the link and QR code at the end of this chapter.

1LT Mark Bashaw was also retaliated against for doing his job. He was "restricted from his place of duty," had his security access to certain health facilities suspended, threatened with imprisonment and "convicted" in a court-martial, though he was sentenced to no further punishment. Callender explained that "the judge even recommended to the commanding general to drop the findings of the court martial in whole." Instead, the judge initiated proceedings for involuntary separation of 1LT Bashaw from the military, but this soldier continues to fight against this lawlessness.

An article in late March 2022 reported on the case seeking an injunction against the military vaccine mandate (Seals 1 v Austin).[212] Four military medical doctors, including LTC Long and LTC Chambers, testified in support of the injunction. However, the Department of Defense offered no witnesses in any of the three hearings that had been held up to that time, despite the judge urging the DoD to do so. **Why not?**

Comments by the plaintiffs' attorney, Mat Staver of Liberty Counsel, answer that question.[213] He told reporter Daniel Horowitz that the information the DOD had been presenting in court is "'outdated, wrong and would really be subject to dismantling under cross examination.'" He also stated that cross examination of his witnesses "only made their case stronger." Not only that, but the judge told the DOD lawyers that they had "a frail case," and were "acting as though they were above the law."

Perhaps the most alarming testimony came from LTC Long in response to questions posed by her attorney, as reported earlier, where she repeatedly stated that she had been ordered not to answer. When Judge Merryday demanded to know who was ordering her not to testify, she disclosed that she had been ordered the night before by her command not to testify about any military data. Her attorney said that would be considered witness tampering. LTC Long also testified that she feared for the life and safety of her family and children.[214]

Her attorney then asked if the information she was ordered to withhold was "relevant and helpful for the court and the public to know." When she said "yes," and the attorney asked why, she explained:

DEVASTATING IMPACTS ON THE MILITARY

"'**I have so many soldiers being destroyed by this vaccine**. Not a single member of my senior command has discussed my concerns with me ... I have nothing to gain and everything to lose by talking about it. I'm OK with that because *I am watching people get absolutely destroyed.*'"

With regard to the impact of the vaccine mandates on national security, Callender shared the following portion of LTC Long's testimony:

"the impact of the relentless coercion, intimidation, threats, abuse of authority and blatant disregard for bodily autonomy and religious freedom, has directly resulted in devastation to medical and force readiness, in the form of failed recruiting, retention, mass resignation and forced separation of personal that hold critical military occupational specialties - in addition to attrition from vaccine-induced medical injury."

The DOD's conduct speaks volumes. Among other things: 1) ignoring a military doctor's concerns about the serious injuries from the shots, and ordering her to not to talk about vaccine injuries; 2) court-martialing a preventive medicine officer for doing his job of reporting health risks based on the military database; 3) altering data after being advised by a U.S. Senator to preserve the evidence; and 4) ordering a witness to withhold information. By the time you finish Part 4 of this book, you will understand what is behind the DOD's actions.

---

[198] Todd Callender is the principal in the law firm Disabled Rights Advocates PLLC and is the CEO of a large health & disability insurance group based in Colorado.

[199] Robert v. Austin, Civil Action No. 21-CV-2228 filed Aug. 17, 2021 in the U.S. Federal District Court for the District of Colorado, https://ia904609.us.archive.org/23/items/gov.uscourts.cod.209086/gov.uscourts.cod.209086.1.0.pdf

[200] Information told to Sally Saxon by Todd Callender, Nov. 2022, https://www.sallysaxon.com/covid-19-vax-military-whistleblower-documents

[201] https://renz-law.com/that-will-be-used-to-cover-the-death-of-children-from-the-covid-shot/

[202] In a letter dated February 8, 2022 from Sen. Ron Johnson, to Secretary of Defense Lloyd Austin, referring to his January 24, 2022 letter, https://www.ronjohnson.senate.gov/services/files/07514E29-F80B-4EB6-B0F4-D7156A8C5691

203 https://renz-law.com/that-will-be-used-to-cover-the-death-of-children-from-the-covid-shot/
204 Letter dated Feb.1, 2022 to Secretary Lloyd Austin, Dept. of the Defense, https://www.ronjohnson.senate.gov/services/files/FB6DDD42-4755-4FDC-BEE9-50E402911E02
205 DonG, https://ricochet.com/1127182/dmed-is-a-game-changer-on-vaccine-safety/ (Feb. 27, 2022)
206 Communication from Todd Callender to Sally Saxon, Nov. 2022,
207 https://www.politifact.com/factchecks/2022/jan/31/instagram-posts/numbers-were-based-faulty-data-military-spokespers/ (Jan. 28, 2022)
208 Letter dated February 8, 2022 from Sen. Ron Johnson, to Secretary Lloyd Austin
209 Declaration of 1LT Mark Bashaw in Further Support of Senator Ron Johnson's Investigation into the Safety and Efficacy of COVID-19 Vaccines, March 3, 2022. https://takeactionforfreedom.com/docs/1LT%20Mark%20Bashaw%20Whistleblower%20Declaration.pdf
210 Communication from Todd Callender to Sally Saxon, Nov. 2022,
211 Declaration of LTC Theresa Long, MD, MPH, FA in Further Support of Senator Ron Johnson's Investigation into the Safety and Efficacy of COVID-19 Vaccines (March 9, 2022), https://www.sallysaxon.com/covid-19-vax-military-whistleblower-documents, p. 20
212 https://ac.news/military-doctor-testifies-she-was-ordered-to-cover-up-vaccine-injuries/(March 31, 2022); https://en-volve.com/2022/03/30/military-doctor-testifies-under-oath-that-she-was-ordered-to-cover-up-vaccine-injuries-through-biden-admin-directive/ (March 30, 2022)
213 Id.
214 Id.

To access LTC Theresa Long's March 9, 2022 Declaration, other military whistleblower affidavits and related whistleblower information, go to SallySaxon.com or use this QR code.

Chapter 14
Data for Those 65 and Older

Data compiled by a whistleblower from the CMS database (Center for Medicare and Medicaid Services) was provided to attorney Thomas Renz. It shows that among *the Medicare population alone*, as of mid-2021, only about half a year after the vaccine rollout, there were **over 50,000 deaths within 14 days of the 1st or 2nd shot**.[215] What might the current number be? In fact, compare that number with the VAERS number as of August 12, 2022, *more than a year later*, which showed only 14,081 U.S. deaths for ALL age groups following the COVID shots. Somebody's numbers are way off.

Analyzing data directly from the CMS database, the whistleblower found that 555 people died the day of the first shot. Among those who survived long enough to get the 2nd shot, another 329 died the same day they got that one. The day after each shot, another 1,137 and 1,023 died, respectively. Except for day 11 after the 2nd shot, each day within the first 14 days after either shot, the number of deaths increased steadily.

Some of those 50,000+ may well have died anyway from other causes within the 2-week period after their shots. But consider this: *if a person were in such poor condition that they were not likely to live longer than a couple weeks or even a few months due to comorbidities, do you think they would even have bothered to get the shot?* It is not likely. *What would have been the point, if death were fairly imminent anyway?*

Therefore, it is reasonable to suggest that those age 65+ who did get the shot – even if they had various comorbidities – were not likely to die from their other conditions any time soon. Therefore, the fact that there were so many deaths within just a two-week period reflects a strong causal connection between their death and the COVID vaccines.

Renz stated in an interview with Stew Peters that **because those 50,000 deaths all occurred within 14 days of injection, they were all counted as deaths of "unvaccinated" persons. That is because of the CDC's very** *misleading definition of "vaccinated."*[216] To be counted as vaccinated for this purpose, according to the CDC, a person had to have been "fully vaccinated" *14 or more day*s earlier. (See more about this 14-day definition below.)

Another study of this older group was done by Dr. Ronald N. Kostoff, Ph.D. and his team using the VAERS data.[217] (This paper was later retracted, but see the brief discussion below about the reasons for the retraction.) The number of deaths for this demographic at that time in VAERS was substantially smaller than the numbers from the CMS database, due to the different ways the data is collected for those databases. They did "a non-traditional *best-case scenario* pseudo-cost-benefit analysis of the COVID-19 inoculations for the 65+ demographic in the USA." The results refute FDA findings that the benefits of these shots outweigh the risks:

> "our extremely conservative estimate for risk-benefit ratio is about 5/1. In plain English, people in the 65+ demographic are five times as likely to die from the inoculation as from COVID-19 under the most favorable assumptions!"

The paper even goes so far as to suggest a URF that is consistent with that of VAERS expert Albert Benavides discussed above:

> "Thus, based on the deaths reported in VAERS following COVID-19 inoculation, and assuming the inoculation-related deaths are reported in the same ratio as expected deaths, the actual number of deaths strongly related to the COVID-19 inoculation should be scaled up by factors of 100 - 200."

The Kostoff paper was later retracted at the request of the Founding Editor Prof. Lawrence H. Lash. Its findings were alleged to be "unreliable" due to "inappropriate bias in multiple ways." After reading the specific allegations mentioned, it appears that this retraction was made simply because the paper is contrary to the official narrative. The reasons cited actually reveal "inappropriate bias" *on the part of the retractor*. For example, he said: "The use of … the key terms 'inoculation' and 'vaccination' diverges from common use … indicating clear evidence of bias." This is referring to statements in the article similar to ones in Part 1 of this book as to why the COVID shots are not true "vaccines" – because they do not meet the traditional or legal definitions of a vaccine. For that reason, Kostoff and his team used the word "inoculations" instead. This terminology change was alleged to show bias. *However, based on the traditional and legal definitions presented in Part 1, is it not actually the CDC's definition and use of the word "vaccine" that "diverges from common use?"*

Another point of alleged "bias" dealt with alleged misinterpretation of CDC data. Interestingly, the statements in question were *statements on the CDC's own website, but they happen to reveal an "inconvenient truth" that greatly undermines the official narrative.* This is another example of the serious bias of the so-called "fact-checkers" and why they need to be fact-checked themselves.

With regard to *COVID deaths* in the 65+ age group, attorney Tom Renz also pointed out that the government database showed that **60% were among fully vaccinated people.** Stew Peters added that his staff checked the source of that data a bit later and found that **the figure had increased to 70%.** The question arises, however, whether all of the deaths reported as COVID were actually COVID deaths, or whether many may have been vaccine-related deaths.

---

[215] https://renz-law.com/special-notice-regarding-evidentiary-findings-related-to-the-official-renz-law-covid-19-investigation/, pp. 156-157

[216] Tom Renz interviewed by Stew Peters, https://www.bitchute.com/video/ETn60yF7CNFt/ (Oct. 4, 2021)

[217] Ronald N. Kostoff, PhD, et al, "Why are We Vaccinating Children Against COVID-19?" https://www.sciencedirect.com/science/article/pii/S221475002100161X#bib002(2021)

Chapter 15
Dangers of Giving COVID Shots to Children

Thousands of doctors all over the world have strongly warned against giving the COVID shots to children, and data for children who have received the shots reveal why. Dr. Daniel Nagase, the Canadian doctor cited earlier, analyzed the Pfizer report of data through February 28, 2021 with respect to children.[218] He noted 34 instances where children under 12 were given this injection between December 2020 and February 28, 2021. Dr. Jessica Rose's first question was: *why were any children under 12 even given this injection, since it had not been authorized for them at that point?*[219] Of those 34, twenty-four had serious side effects, and of those, 13 had not resolved, 16 had resolved or were resolving, and 5 were unknown. Thirteen of 34 had a non-resolving side effect, which is almost 40%. In Dr. Nagase's opinion, the data in Pfizer's own report shows why **these injections absolutely should not be given to children**. He elaborated further with regard to the very serious and damaging effects that mRNA can have in the cells of children who are still developing.

Remember the information from the casket manufacturer referred to in Part 1 who said that their business actually ***decreased*** by about 60% in 2020.[220] He has also stated that for the first time in their company's 30+ year history, they have started to get *bulk orders* for child caskets. He stated that before the vaccine rollout, they would get about 1 child casket order for every 5 full-size ones. After the vaccines started being given to children, he estimated that the ratio changed to about 2 child casket orders for every 5 full-size orders. However, the increase he reported in a different interview in July 2022, in terms of actual numbers, is even more chilling. He first noted that "all casket sales are up dramatically in the last two years" (since 2021) because "something is happening that is causing an unprecedented amount of deaths." When he was asked how many caskets were in a bulk order (referring to child caskets), his response was: "If we went through an average of, say 50-60 a year, the last order was

200 and the next order after that was 250." He added: "We've now basically sold 5 years' worth of stock in 7 months."[221] (That statistic is even worse than that if the total of those last two orders, 450, were both in the last 7 months, rather than just 250.) *And yet we are told that these shots are safe and effective for children as young as 6 months old.*

The results of a CDC survey of more than 13,000 infants and toddlers was released September 1, 2022. They showed that more than 55% of the children had "systemic reactions" (reactions beyond the injection site) following their first Pfizer COVID shot, and almost 60% had such a reaction to their second dose of Moderna. Six percent (or about 780) of the children were reported to be "unable to do normal activities" after their second dose. [222]

At least one state has refused to go along with the official federal level recommendations. A Guidance statement issued by the State of Florida in March 2022 recommended *against* COVID vaccines for healthy children and adolescents ages 5 through 17. It later extended this recommendation against COVID vaccines to infants and children under 5 after an EUA had been granted for that age group.[223]

An article dated September 2022 reports various statistics based on official data from Europe for children following authorization of the COVID shots for children ages 5-11 and 12-15.[224] All showed alarming increases in excess deaths following the vaccine rollouts, compared with baseline averages from previous years. The vaccine rollouts for 12 to 15-year-olds was May 28, 2021 (week 22) and Nov. 25, 2021 for 5 to 11-year-olds. Among the many statistics and charts reported in that article are:

- **691% increase in excess deaths of children 0-14,** starting week 22 of 2021 up to week 33 of 2022 (total of 1,856) compared with the average (234.75) from week 22 in 2017 up to week 33 of 2021.

- **381% increase in excess deaths among children** in the 1st 33 weeks of 2022 (total 841) compared with the annual average of 174 excess deaths for the 1st 33 weeks in baseline years 2018-2021

An interview with Dr. Claire Craig, a diagnostic pathologist, has exposed the manipulation in the clinical trial data underlying the FDA's authorization of Pfizer's COVID shots for the 6-months through four-year-olds.[225] There were originally 4,526 children in this trial, but 3,000, or 2/3 of them did not make it to the end. ***Why not? What happened to them?*** That unanswered question alone, according to Dr. Craig, should have rendered the trial results that the FDA relied on null and void, until there was a satisfactory answer to that question. ***If it was because most of them had serious adverse reactions, think of how that would skew the results if they were not accounted for in the final data, and how that would affect parents' decisions for their children.***

If parents knew how this approval came about, it is doubtful they would want their children to get these shots. There was much in this trial that shocked her. It seems that Pfizer ignored many trial data that were not in its favor. In all, ***she said they ignored 97% of it!*** In the end, she reported, they focused on 3 vaccinated children who got COVID and 7 in the placebo group. It was on that basis, she said, the vaccine was deemed effective.

Dr. Eric Rubin is an adjunct professor of immunology and infectious diseases at Harvard University and editor-in-chief of the *New England Journal of Medicine*. He also sat on the FDA advisory committee that decided 17-0 to recommend approval of the Pfizer COVID vaccine for 5-11-year-olds. During a committee meeting, he made the statement: **"We're never going to learn how safe this vaccine is unless we start giving it."** [226] ***Is that an admission that the clinical trials were essentially useless and could not establish that the vaccines were safe as the public was being told?***

The "fact-checker" *Politifact* tried to explain that comment was taken out of context by many alleged "misinformation spreaders." Rubin acknowledged that with regard to youth, they [the committee members] were more concerned about side effects, because the benefit of the vaccine for youth was not as large as with adults. ***He noted that the side effect they were concerned about was myocarditis, which studies showed there was an increased risk of, particularly in male adolescents.*** However, he said that according to the CDC, myocarditis cases "have tended to be clinically mild."

Rubin's statement was made in late October, 2021 and FDA authorized the Pfizer shots for 5 to 11-year-olds shortly thereafter. As of April 1, 2022, data show a **17,495% increase** in the monthly average for "carditis" cases in children under 18 after COVID vaccinations, compared with monthly averages of "carditis" cases published in VAERS from all other vaccines over 30 years.[227] VAERS data for the period from December 14, 2020, to July 29,

2022 reveals 1,292 reports of myocarditis and pericarditis for the 12 to 17-year-old age group following COVID vaccination, of which 1,145 involved the Pfizer shots.[228]

Remember that a URF needs to be applied to get a much more accurate estimate of the number of cases. Steve Kirsch's older and much more conservative estimated URF of 41 would yield almost 53,000 cases, as of July 29, 2022. The higher URF that Benavides believes is more accurate, given additional factors since Kirsch's original URF calculations, would mean that there are about 129,200 cases.

Table 13 below shows data published in VAERS for 5 to 11 and 12 to 17-year-olds from Dec. 14, 2020 to July 29, 2022, as reported by the Children's Health Defense organization just for the U.S. (and U.S. territories and 'unknown"), and what a more realistic number would be if a URF of only 41 were applied:[229]

Table 13. VAERS data, Dec. 14, 2020 to July 29, 2022 for 5 to 17-year-olds (for the "U.S., Territories or Unknown")

Type of AE	5-11 y.o.	12-17 y.o.	Total	If a URF of 41 is applied
Total AEs reported	12,379	32,910	45,289	1,856,849
AEs reported as serious	315	1,850	2,165	88,765
Deaths	9	45	54	2,214
Myocarditis/pericarditis	24	658*	682	27,962
Bloodclotting disorders	47	165**	212	8,692

* Pfizer shots accounted for 645 of the 658.   ** Pfizer shots account for all 165

According to cardiologist Dr. Peter McCullough, a 2022 preprint study in Thailand [230] of 13 to 18-year-olds was the first prospective cohort study, one which the FDA had asked the manufacturers to do, but they did not, nor did any of the major universities.[231] It was left to come first out of Thailand. This study showed that 18% of 301 teens who were healthy and showed no abnormal symptoms after their first Pfizer dose *had an abnormal EKG after their second dose.*[232] McCullough also noted that the study showed that ***29% of the teens had some cardiovascular symptoms.***[233] In addition, 3.5% of the young men in the study "developed myopericarditis or subclinical myocarditis, two were hospitalized and one was admitted to the ICU for heart problems."[234] McCullough was alarmed by the data suggesting that so many vaccinated children could be developing heart issues. Dr. Tracy Høeg, MD, Ph.D., an epidemiologist, described the study as "'unique & impressive because of the extensive workup both pre and post vaccination...'" [235] Those workups included EKGs, echocardiograms and cardiac enzymes to determine if any changes occurred in the participants' cardiac conditions.

McCullough was especially concerned about the study's finding that some have heart damage without even knowing it because they had no symptoms yet.[236] He was concerned because heart damage causes scarring which is a "setup for an abnormal heart rhythm," and that, in turn, can lead to cardiac arrest. "The reason why myocarditis is so important in children is that when there's superimposed adrenaline and noradrenaline in exercise, it is the trigger for cardiac arrest." McCullough added that could also explain why so many athletes have collapsed or died on the field. (See the chapter on athlete data below.)

McCullough had other important insights about myocarditis from this study. In one interview he did around the time that Washington, DC announced a vaccine mandate for children, he lamented that some of those children were "going to sustain heart damage and they don't know it. And they'll only find out later if it results in sudden death or heart failure."[237]

He also noted that the baseline rate for myocarditis, before COVID, was 4 cases/million, and that the CDC has said that after the vaccines were introduced, it rose to 62/million. The CDC website accessed in mid-September, 2022[238] states that for the period from December 2020 – August 2021, "CDC scientists found that rates of myocarditis were highest following the second dose of an mRNA vaccine among males in the following age groups:

- 12–15 years (70.7 cases per one million doses of Pfizer-BioNTech)
- 16–17 years (105.9 cases per one million doses of Pfizer-BioNTech)"

McCullough went on to say that Kaiser-Permanente has said the rate is about 500/million, but now, after this first prospective study in Thailand,

DANGERS OF GIVING COVID SHOTS TO CHILDREN

McCullough said the *rate for myocarditis is probably about 25,000 cases/million.*[239] That will include a large number of children.

Strong Warnings Against the Shots for Children. Surprisingly, even the World Health Organization stated in January of 2022 that children under 12 "should not be routinely vaccinated" against COVID, noting the lack of safety and efficacy data.[240] It advised governments to hold off giving these vaccines to children on the grounds there was no safety and efficacy data to support their use for that group.

In a short 5-minute video, Dr. Robert Malone has also emphatically warned against children getting the COVID vaccines.[241] He concludes that "the risk/benefit analysis isn't even close," for three main reasons.

> *"The first is that a viral gene will be injected into your children's cells. This gene forces your child's body to make toxic spike proteins. These proteins often cause permanent damage in children's critical organs, including their brain and nervous system, their heart and blood vessels, including blood clots, their reproductive system and this vaccine can trigger fundamental changes to their immune system. The most alarming point... once these damages have occurred, they are irreparable...*
>
> *"The second thing you need to know about is the fact that this novel technology has not been adequately tested. We need at least 5 years of testing/research before we... understand the risks. Harms and risks from new medicines often become revealed many years later. Ask yourself if you want your own child to be part of the most radical medical experiment in human history.*
>
> *"One final point: the reason they're giving you to vaccinate your child is a lie... children represent no danger to their parents or grandparents. It's actually the opposite... there is no benefit ... to be vaccinating your children against the small risks of the virus, given the known health risks of the vaccine that as a parent, you and your children may have to live with for the rest of their lives."*

Rome Declaration. As of January 18, 2022, over 17,000 physicians and scientists all over the world had signed the Rome Declaration.[242] That group recognized "the imminent threat to humanity brought forth by current Covid-19 policies." It stated the following conclusions with regard to children:

> 1) there were "negligible clinical risks of SARS-CoV-2 infection" among healthy children
>
> 2) the long-term effects of the shots could not be determined;
>
> 3) children risked severe adverse events from these shots. "Permanent physical damage to the brain, heart, immune and reproductive system associated with SARS-CoV-2 spike protein-based genetic vaccines has been demonstrated in children."
>
> 4) "Healthy unvaccinated children are critical to achieving herd immunity."

Ninety-three Israeli doctors sent "a joint letter of protest calling to refrain from administering Covid-19 vaccines to children." The doctors said: "Do not rush to vaccinate children as long as the full picture is not clear. Coronavirus disease does not endanger children..." [243] They also wrote:

> "'it cannot be ruled out that the vaccine will have long-term adverse effects that have not yet been discovered at this time, including on growth, reproductive system or fertility. Children should be allowed a quick return to routine; the many tests and broad isolation cycles should be stopped, and no separation between the vaccinated and unvaccinated should be created....'"

The Canadian COVID Care Alliance wrote a guide to help parents decide about the shots for their kids. It then appealed to the government: "The Canadian government should ... immediately halt the mass vaccination program of children and adolescents until such time as these studies are conducted and the uncertainties about the potential pathogenicity of the spike protein can be addressed." [244] The Kostoff study[245] discussed above (the one that was retracted), entitled "*Why are We Vaccinating Children Against COVID-19?*" advises that **"mass inoculation of children 12–15 years old based on the trials ... cannot be justified on any cost-benefit ratio findings."** It appears that the younger the child, the higher the rate of adverse reactions.

Despite all the warnings, Anthony Fauci has suggested that kids 2 to 5 years old should probably get a regimen of three COVID shots.[246] And the

FDA has now authorized children as young as six-month old babies to get the COVID shots. [247] *Parents and doctors, are you okay with this?*

---

[218] Interview on Strong and Free Truthcast https://rumble.com/vqq3hw-breaking-news-pfizers-own-stats-1200-40000-trial-participants-dead-intervie.html (Dec. 13, 2021)

[219] https://jessicar.substack.com/p/pfizer-adverse-event-data (Dec. 5 2021)

[220] Miranda Sellick, https://rairfoundation.com/coffins-for-children-ordered-in-bulk-first-time-in-over-30-years-exclusive-interview/ (July 14, 2022)

[221] Mick Haddock interviewed by Stew Peters, https://rumble.com/v1bwqm3-casket-salesman-blows-whistle-child-caskets-being-ordered-in-bulk-never-see.html (July 11, 2022)

[222] Margaret Menge, https://www.theepochtimes.com/more-than-half-of-babies-toddlers-surveyed-had-systemic-reaction-after-covid-19-vaccine_4707948.html (Sept. 4, 2022)

[223] https://floridahealthcovid19.gov/wp-content/uploads/2022/10/20221007-guidance-mrna-covid19-vaccines-doc.pdf

[224] https://expose-news.com/2022/09/13/urope-children-killed-covid-vaccine/?cmid=bad6ac5f-965f-4b03-8cf2-ed9383ba44f4 (Sept. 13, 2022)

[225] Dr. Claire Craig interviewed by Del Bigtree, https://thehighwire.com/videos/how-did-the-covid-vaccine-get-approved-for-kids/ (June 28, 2022) ; Dr. Claire Craig, https://rumble.com/v1ah75c-dr.-claire-craig-how-the-fda-twisted-the-data-6-month-to-4-year-olds.html (June 29, 2022)

[226] Tom Kerthcher, https://www.politifact.com/article/2021/nov/01/context-never-going-learn-how-safe-vaccine-unless-/ (Nov. 1, 2021)

[227] https://healthimpactnews.com/2022/17500-increase-in-heart-disease-in-children-following-covid-19-vaccines-this-is-not-rare/ (April 2, 2022)

[228] Megan Redshaw, https://childrenshealthdefense.org/defender/pfizer-covid-vaccine-myocarditis-teens-study/ (Aug. 11, 2022)

[229] Megan Redshaw, https://childrenshealthdefense.org/defender/17-year-old-died-myocarditis-pfizer-shot-vaers-data/ (Aug. 5, 2022)

[230] Mansanguan, S.; Charunwatthana, P. et al. Cardiovascular Manifestation of the BNT162b2 mRNA COVID-19 Vaccine in Adolescents. Trop. Med. Infect. Dis.2022, 7, 196. https://doi.org/10.3390/tropicalmed7080196

[231] Dr. Peter McCullough interviewed by Nadera Lopez-Garrity, https://childrenshealthdefense.org/video-post/new-generation-of-covid-19-shots-what-you-must-know-with-dr-peter-mccullough/ (Sept. 5, 2022)

[232] Megan Redshaw, https://childrenshealthdefense.org/defender/pfizer-covid-vaccine-myocarditis-teens-study/ (Aug. 11, 2022)

[233] Dr. Peter McCullough interviewed by Nadera Lopez-Garrity, https://childrenshealthdefense.org/video-post/new-generation-of-covid-19-shots-what-you-must-know-with-dr-peter-mccullough/ (Sept. 5, 2022)

[234] Megan Redshaw, https://childrenshealthdefense.org/defender/pfizer-covid-vaccine-myocarditis-teens-study/ (Aug. 11, 2022)

[235] Id.

[236] Dr. Peter McCullough interviewed by Kim Iversen, https://www.alipac.us/f19/dr-peter-mccullough-discusses-number-vaccinated-children-developing-subclinical-m-398396/; https://rumble.com/embed/v1d9dyz/?pub=4 (Aug 14. 2022)

[237] Dr. Peter McCullough interviewed by Nadera Lopez-Garrity, https://childrenshealthdefense.org/video-post/new-generation-of-covid-19-shots-what-you-must-know-with-dr-peter-mccullough/ (Sept. 5, 2022)

[238] https://www.cdc.gov/coronavirus/2019-ncov/vaccines/safety/adverse-events.html

[239] Dr. Peter McCullough interviewed by Nadera Lopez-Garrity, https://childrenshealthdefense.org/video-post/new-generation-of-covid-19-shots-what-you-must-know-with-dr-peter-mccullough/ (Sept. 5, 2022)

[240] Jack Bingham, https://www.lifesitenews.com/news/children-under-12-should-not-risk-receiving-pfizers-covid-vaccine-who-says/ (Jan. 20, 2022)

[241] https://rwmalonemd.substack.com/p/the-continued-damages-to-our-children

[242] https://doctorsandscientistsdeclaration.org/

[243] https://www.israelnationalnews.com/news/304124 (April 11, 2021)

[244] https://www.lifesitenews.com/wp-content/uploads/2021/06/2021-05-31_-_Guide_to_COVID-19_vaccines_for_parents_-_FINAL.pdf

[245] Ronald N. Kostoff, PhD, et al, "Why are We Vaccinating Children Against COVID-19?" ,https://www.sciencedirect.com/science/article/pii/S221475002100161X#bib002 (2021)

[246] Jack Phillips, https://www.theepochtimes.com/fauci-looks-like-children-aged-4-and-younger-will-get-a-three-dose-vaccine-regimen_4240317.html (Jan. 27, 2022)

[247] Manas Mishra and Michael Erman, https://news.yahoo.com/u-fda-panel-weighs-covid-110649297.html (June 15, 2022)

Chapter 16
Adverse Impacts on Athletes

One of the most telling pieces of evidence is the staggering number of young healthy athletes collapsing after the COVID vaccine rollout, mostly during training or competitions, even though they are among the most fit and healthy people in society. The International Olympic Committee studied data from 1966 to 2004 and found an average of 29 deaths per year worldwide of athletes under 35 years old.[248] However, between the COVID vaccine rollout and mid-November 2022, at least 1,502 athletes have collapsed, of whom 1,029 have died.[249] In the vaccine's first 20 months (1.66 years), that is an annual average of 510 athlete deaths, which is an increase of nearly 18X or 1,800%.

As much as many doctors only pay attention to data from randomized double-blinded, placebo-controlled clinical trials, athletic coaches who get paid to observe the performance of their athletes are in a position to know when their athletes are not performing up to their own previous levels, and how they compare with other athletes. Their observations, together with their knowledge of each athlete's "baseline" performance, can serve a similar purpose as VAERS, as an early warning system that something is not right. This is especially true if there are similar declines in performance among multiple athletes around the same time, and the common denominator among them was that they all had received the COVID vaccine, while unvaccinated athletes suffered no such declines.

In her book, *Neither Safe Nor Effective: The Evidence Against the COVID Vaccines,* Dr. Colleen Huber reports on her interviews with two sports coaches who each worked with a group of 20 student athletes.[250] Fifteen were high school age and the rest were younger. The students had spoken openly and freely about their vaccination status, and how they felt after receiving the shots. Half were vaccinated, and half were not. The coaches had to speak under conditions of anonymity, for obvious reasons. The coaches found the following: with regard to the vaccinated students:

- None were competing at their own previous levels, and were even worse than in 2020.
- None demonstrated their previous endurance during exercise drills.
- Recovery times were longer than before, and longer compared to the other students.
- Most or all complained of at least one of the following: "a) chest pain; b) dizziness; c) seeing stars; d) feeling faint; and e) shortness of breath;"
- "Unvaccinated girls are now beating vaccinated boys in a competition, whom they could not do well against last year."
- Most of the above symptoms were still evident in all of the vaccinated athletes even several months later

Unvaccinated students did not experience any of the above symptoms or declines in their performance or endurance, but continued to improve. According to Huber, the above information came solely from spontaneous remarks by the students themselves, with no prompting from the coaches as to symptoms they were experiencing.

---

[248] Bille K, Figueiras D, Schamasch P, Kappenberger L, et al. Sudden cardiac death in athletes: the Lausanne Recommendations. Eur J Cardiovasc Prev Rehabil. 2006 Dec;13(6):859-75. doi: 10.1097/01.hjr.0000238397.50341.4a. PMID: 17143117; https://pubmed.ncbi.nlm.nih.gov/17143117/

[249] https://goodsciencing.com/covid/athletes-suffer-cardiac-arrest-die-after-covid-shot/ (data showing in headline when accessed Aug. 15, 2022)

[250] Dr. Colleen Huber, NMD, *Neither Safe Nor Effective: The Evidence Against the COVID Vaccines*, (2022) pp. 79-84

Chapter 17
Dangers of the Spike Protein

It is well-known that mRNA vaccines produce spike proteins. The way mRNA vaccines are supposed to work is explained on the CDC website:[251]

> "mRNA vaccines use mRNA created in a laboratory to teach our cells how to make a protein—or even just a piece of a protein—that triggers an immune response inside our bodies. That immune response, which produces antibodies, is what protects us from getting infected if the real virus enters our bodies."

The CDC website also says that scientists estimate that the spike protein might stay in the body up to a few weeks, and that the spike protein is "harmless." However, both of these claims have been shown not to be true, as discussed below.

Before the discussion of the various dangers of the spike protein, consider some important comments by Dr. Michael Yeadon, a former Pfizer V.P. and chief scientist, about the manufacturers' choice of the spike protein as a primary feature of these "vaccines." In an interview in June 2022,[252] Yeadon explained why it was a poor choice on which to base the COVID shots: 1) it was known to be toxic; 2) it produced an inferior immune response compared with other parts of the virus; 3) it mutates too rapidly to be very effective; and 4) it is also "similar to a variety of human proteins, which can trigger your body to mount an inappropriate immune response against your own proteins. In other words, it can cause autoimmune disease." He said that about 90% of the immune response a person gets from natural COVID infection is in response to other parts of the virus, not the spike protein. To sum it up, Yeadon said that the choice of the spike protein "violated all of the accepted rules for creating a safe and effective product." Yet the scientists chose it anyway, and not just from one manufacturer, but all of them. That is a point that Yeadon comments further on in another context.

The America's Frontline Doctors group, which has been in the forefront of providing early treatment using proven highly effective protocols, prepared a report entitled *"Identifying Post-Vaccination Complications and Their Causes: An Analysis of COVID-19 Patient Data."* It states:

> "There are two major neurological concerns related to the COVID vaccines. These are the spike proteins and the lipid nanoparticles which carry the mRNA into the cell. They are both capable of passing through the 'blood-brain barrier' which typically keeps the brain and spinal cord completely insulated from entrants into the body. There simply has not been enough time to know what brain problems and how often a brain problem will develop from that. There is concern amongst many scientists for prion disease (neurodegenerative brain disease).
>
> "Traditional vaccines do not pass through the blood-brain barrier. Crossing the blood-brain barrier places patients at risk of chronic inflammation and thrombosis (clotting) in the neurological system, contributing to tremors, chronic lethargy, stroke, Bell's Palsy and ALS-type symptoms. The lipid nanoparticles can potentially fuse with brain cells, resulting in delayed neuro-degenerative disease. And the mRNA-induced spike protein can bind to brain tissue 10 to 20 times stronger than the spike proteins that are (naturally) part of the original virus."[253]

An article entitled "The Killer in the Bloodstream: the 'Spike Protein'" (published in June 2021) sheds more light on this subject.[254] It summarizes the findings of a study by the Salk Institute:[255]

> "Salk researchers and collaborators show how the protein damages cells, ***confirming COVID-19 as a primarily vascular disease*** ... SARS-CoV-2 virus damages and attacks the vascular system ... on a cellular level... scientists studying other coronaviruses have long suspected that the spike protein contributed to damaging vascular endothelial cells, but this is the first time the process has been documented....
>
> ... the spike protein alone was enough to cause disease. ... 'If you remove the replicating capabilities of the virus, it still has a major damaging effect on the vascular cells, simply by virtue of its ability to bind to this ACE2 receptor, the S protein receptor...'"

Dr. Byram Bridle is a viral immunologist and associate professor at University of Guelph, Ontario who was awarded a government grant for research on COVID vaccine development. In an interview in May 2021, Dr. Bridle explained that he was very much pro-vaccine, but that he and others had just discovered some new pieces of information that enabled them to understand the problems they were seeing after the COVID vaccines. He explained: [256]

> "'One of these is that the spike protein, on its own, is almost entirely responsible for the damage to the cardiovascular system, if it gets into circulation. Indeed, if you inject the purified spike protein into the blood of research animals they get all kinds of damage to the cardiovascular system, and it can cross the blood-brain barrier and cause damage to the brain.'"

He said that at first they were not concerned about that because they were injecting into the shoulder muscle. They assumed that just like with traditional vaccines, these vaccines would also stay in the shoulder, though some of the protein would go into the lymph nodes to activate the immune system. But then he and other international collaborators obtained a copy of the biodistribution study for Pfizer by Japanese researchers.[257]

He said it was the first time that scientists had been able to see where the mRNA vaccines actually go in the body after injection. They discovered their assumption was wrong about the vaccine staying in the shoulder. Actually, the spike protein gets into the blood and circulates over several days after vaccination. The big danger is that "the lipid nanoparticles containing the mRNA accumulate in almost every organ of the body, *particularly the ovaries*."[258] Bridle acknowledged: *"We made a big mistake. We didn't realize it until now... that* **by vaccinating people we are inadvertently inoculating them with a toxin.** In some people this gets into the circulation; and when that happens, in some people it can cause damage, especially to the cardiovascular system."

According to Dr. Michael Yeadon, **the manufacturers have known since at least 2012 that the lipid nanoparticles circulate all over the body and accumulate in the organs, especially in the brain and ovaries.** [259] **When did the CDC and FDA first know this? Where are their warnings to the public and to medical professionals?**

Another issue is that no one knows how long it actually stays in the body and continues manufacturing spike protein. Yeadon describes the lack of proper testing to determine this ahead of time as a "catastrophic failure" on the part of the regulatory agencies.[260] One study shows that it was still present at the end of a 15-month long study.[261] According to Dr. Paul Alexander, that "means that if each injection that introduces spike will result in spike and components remaining in the blood for 15 months, then by that timeline, it will take many years to clear spike out of the blood stream. How would the body or does the body react to this? Was our immune system set up for this?"[262]

Particular Concerns About the Spike Protein's Effects on Fertility

Many doctors have become concerned about the biodistribution study's findings, especially with regard to fertility in both women and men. Yeadon notes that no reproductive toxicology studies were done.[263] He had expressed concern to European officials about potential effects on fertility even before the vaccine rollout: "It must be absolutely ruled out that a vaccine against SARS-CoV-2 could trigger an immune reaction against syncytin-1, as otherwise infertility of indefinite duration could result in vaccinated women." [264] Roxana Bruno, Ph.D. in Immunology, expressed a similar concern: "Because of the similarity between syncytins and the spike protein of SARS-CoV-2, COVID-19 vaccine-induced antibody responses could trigger a cross-reaction against syncytins, causing allergic, cytotoxic and/or autoimmune side effects affecting human health and reproduction." [265]

Yeadon,[266] Dr. James Thorp and others have warned that **NO women of reproductive age should be given these shots.** Thorp explains the reason for this concern is that females have all the gametes they will ever have for life before they are even born, unlike males who can produce millions of sperm per hour throughout their lives. If the ovaries are damaged in any way, that will affect fertility. Dr. Robert Malone expressed the additional concern that *reproductive risks do not always appear in the first generation,* and Dr. Bridle asked: *"will we be rendering young people infertile?"* [267]

Serious infertility issues following the COVID shots have already been documented. After the vaccine rollout, there were "reports of miscarriages and problems seen by fertility clinics where individuals who got the shot had *eggs and sperm that were no longer viable."* [268]

In light of this data, and especially for those who have trouble accepting the possibility that there might be an intentional infertility agenda in connection with a "vaccination program," the film entitled *Infertility: A Diabolical Agenda* provides much food for thought. That documentary was made by award-winning filmmaker Dr. Andy Wakefield, together with executive producer Robert F Kennedy, Jr. and Children's Health Defense Films.[269] It premiered in June 2022, and "exposes a World Health Organization (WHO) population control experiment carried out under the guise of a vaccination program, resulting in the sterilization of women in Africa without their knowledge or consent." ***Could that possibly explain why the medical industrial complex refuses to acknowledge the harm to fertility and continues to promote the COVID shots full steam ahead? Is there some other logical and reasonable explanation why the dangers to fertility are being grossly ignored?***

Related Issues Concerning Women's Menstrual Irregularities

A related issue that affects fertility is the dramatic increase in menstrual abnormalities. As of summer of 2022, VAERS expert Albert Benavides' analysis of the VAERS data showed that this was the most often reported type of adverse reaction following the COVID shots.[270] According to Dr. James Thorp's latest analysis of the data, menstrual abnormalities have increased 1,200-fold since the COVID vaccine rollout.[271]

In the spring of 2021, women by the thousands were sharing their stories of such problems on social media. However, one Facebook group with over 20,000 members was deleted.[272] Social media giants obviously did not want people sharing their stories about post-vaccination problems. That led to others providing a forum for women to share their stories and to do a more detailed analysis of the various kinds of problems females were experiencing after COVID shots. Tiffany Parotto is the Director and Founder of MyCycleStory^{SM} which is an independent study and survey among women who have experienced various kinds of menstrual abnormalities after the COVID vaccine rollout. That survey can be found at the website MyCycleStory.com. The results of the initial survey can be found in an online journal article authored by Parotto, Thorp, et al entitled "COVID-19 and the surge in Decidual Cast Shedding."[273]

That paper acknowledges that "menstrual irregularities increased exponentially starting in 2021." It focused on one type of abnormality known as "decidual cast shedding" (or DCS), in which a large piece of uterine tissue passes from the body in one piece. That paper also states that prior to the COVID vaccine rollout, fewer than 40 cases of decidual cast shedding had been reported in the medical literature over the last 109 years. Following the rollout, 292 cases were reported in only 7.5 months. It is difficult to avoid the suspicion that the vaccines played a significant causative role.

---

[251] https://www.cdc.gov/coronavirus/2019-ncov/vaccines/different-vaccines/mrna.html

[252] https://media.mercola.com/ImageServer/Public/2022/August/PDF/bivalent-covid-vaccine-pdf.pdf (Aug. 22, 2022)

[253] https://americasfrontlinedoctors.org/2/action_alerts/identifying-post-vaccination-complications-their-causes-an-analysis-of-covid-19-patient-data/ (no date)

[254] Mike Whitney, https://www.algora.com/Algora_blog/2021/06/13/the-killer-in-the-bloodstream-the-spike-protein (June 13, 2021)

[255] SARS-CoV-2 Spike Protein Impairs Endothelial Function via Downregulation of ACE 2" by Yuyang Lei, et al, 31 March 2021, *Circulation Research*. DOI: 10.1161/CIRCRESAHA.121.318902

[256] Neville Hodgkinson, "Vaccine scientist: 'We've made a big mistake,'" https://www.conservativewoman.co.uk/vaccine-researcher-weve-made-a-big-mistake/ (June 7, 2021)

[257] Id.

[258] https://www.rodefshalom613.org/2021/06/recently-revealed-japanese-study-shows-covid-vaccines-may-affect-fertility/?utm_source=pocket_mylist

[259] https://www.lifesitenews.com/news/pfizer-vp-vaccination-women-is-stupid-infertility/ (Aug. 19, 2021)

[260] Dr. Michael Yeadon presentation, https://odysee.com/@Quasar:3/Mike-Yeadon-Testimony-for-the-Grand-Jury:9 (testimony date Feb. 4, 2022)

[261] Patterson, Bruce K.; Francisco Edgar B.; Long, Emily; Pise, Amruta; et al, "Persistence of SARS CoV-2 S1 Protein in CD16+ Monocytes in Post-Acute Sequelae of COVID-19 (PASC) Up to 15 Months Post-Infection," bioRxiv 2021.06.25.449905; doi: https://doi.org/10.1101/2021.06.25.449905

[262] Dr. Paul Alexander, https://palexander.substack.com/p/spike-protein-and-components-s-1 (Dec. 12, 2021)

[263] https://www.thelibertybeacon.com/dr-mike-yeadon-continues-as-a-force-for-truth/ (June 7, 2021)

[264] https://www.sott.net/article/445136-Dr-Wodarg-and-Dr-Yeadon-request-a-STOP-of-all-corona-vaccination-studies-due-to-safety-concerns-and-call-for-co-signing-the-petition (Dec. 1, 2020)

[265] https://www.rodefshalom613.org/2021/06/recently-revealed-japanese-study-shows-covid-vaccines-may-affect-fertility/

[266] https://www.sott.net/article/445136-Dr-Wodarg-and-Dr-Yeadon-request-a-STOP-of-all-corona-vaccination-studies-due-to-safety-concerns-and-call-for-co-signing-the-petition (Dec. 1, 2020)

[267] https://www.rodefshalom613.org/2021/06/recently-revealed-japanese-study-shows-covid-vaccines-may-affect-fertility/

[268] Id.

[269] https://childrenshealthdefense.org/press-release/dr-andy-wakefield-and-childrens-health-defense-films-announce-the-premiere-of-infertility-a-diabolical-agenda/ (June 8, 2022)

[270] Communication from Albert Benavides to James A. Thorp and Sally Saxon (Aug.5, 2022)

[271] Communication from James A. Thorp, per his personal analysis of VAERS data. (Aug. 2022)

[272] https://mycyclestory.com/2022/06/25/womens-menstrual-anomalies-lead-to-massive-research-study/

[273] Parotto T, Thorp JA, Hooker B, Mills PJ, Newman J, Murphy L, et al. COVID-19 and the surge in Decidual Cast Shedding. G Med Sci. 2022; 3(1): 107- 117. https://www.doi.org/10.46766/thegms.pubheal.22041401

Chapter 18
The Destructive Impact on the Natural Immune System

One of the biggest issues is evidence that the COVID shots are shutting down and destroying the natural immune system. In order for the lipid nanoparticles (LNPs) and mRNA to survive and not be attacked and inactivated by the recipients' immune system, the vaccine needed to suppress the host's immune system. According to this book's contributing authors, Dr. Deborah Viglione and Dr James A. Thorp, the vaccines are affecting both the innate and adaptive immune system.[274] Some of the known effects so far are: a substitution of uridine for uracil in the bases of the mRNA,[275] suppression of Toll Like Receptors,[276] reduction of CD8 and CD4 T-cells with a vaccine induced acquired immunodeficiency syndrome (VAIDS),[277] increased NF-kB, a reduction of type 1 interferon,[278] reduction in B- cell response,[279] a reduction of p53 expression,[280] and reductions in TNF alpha, and IL1.[281]

Earlier versions of the Moderna website [282] explain that the immune system must be "evaded" for the mRNA to work properly:

> "We need to get the mRNA into the targeted tissue and cells while evading the immune system. If the immune system is triggered, the resultant response may limit protein production and, thus, limit the therapeutic benefit of mRNA medicines."

Pathologist Dr. Ryan Cole confirms that toll-like receptors 3,4,7 and 8 are being "down-regulated after the shots."[283] Cancers have been "taking off like wildfire" because the lipid nanoparticles are shutting down certain pattern receptors, so cancer cells face no opposition.[284]

Attorney Todd Callender, who is also CEO of a large insurance group, has been working with medical and scientific experts who have concluded that the vaccines are destroying people's immune systems.[285] He points to the huge percentages of increases in 2021 in all-cause mortality and morbidity, especially among the military who are the most fit people. As one who is in the "morbidity" business, he says there is only one explanation for this: *their immune systems are being destroyed*. In fact, he also states that "a person's natural immune system has to be disarmed" for the LNPs to deliver their contents, as explained above.

An article in *The Exposé* in May 2022 explains more about this very disturbing problem:

> "Governments worldwide have been quietly publishing data for months on end that strongly suggests the Covid-19 injections cause extensive damage to the natural immune system, causing recipients to develop a new form of Acquired Immunodeficiency Syndrome.
>
> "Now, new data, recently published by the UK's [ONS], indicates that it only takes approximately 4 to 5 months after Covid-19 vaccination, for so much damage to have been done to the immune system that it can, unfortunately, lead to death..." [286]

The founder of the Vaccine Safety Research Foundation, Steve Kirsch, has received data from a whistleblower at HHS (Health and Human Services) that confirm a 5-month interval from vaccination to death for many people, as mentioned in *The Exposé* article just quoted. In his newsletter dated September 1, 2022, Kirsch noted that it has previously been thought that most people who died from the shots died within the first two weeks after vaccination. It is still true that many are dying very quickly.

However, according to his information from the whistleblower, Kirsch states that "most of the deaths from the vaccine are happening an average of 5 months from the last dose [or] the second dose. It may be getting shorter the more shots you get but there are arguments both ways (since there can be survivor bias)." He adds that may be why life insurance companies saw a huge spike in all-cause mortality in the 3rd and 4th quarters of 2021. (That is discussed more in Part 3.) Kirsch also observed that the 5-month delay was "also consistent with death reports where people are developing new aggressive cancers that are killing them over a 4 to 6 months period." This lag time between the last vaccination and death, he notes, is why the causal connection to the vaccine is more difficult to see. However, this correlation appears when an analysis is done on the intervals between dates of death and dates of vaccination and a huge spike at the 5-month mark appears.

In an interview Kirsch did with pathologist Dr. Ryan Cole, Cole stated that **in many cases, the damage done by the shots can only be seen microscopically and therefore does not show up on standardized tests.**[287] That is another reason why medical examiners and other doctors miss the vaccine's causal connection. Information about how to detect vaccine-caused death through autopsies is presented in Part 3.

Kirsch also reports of other mounting evidence that a person's natural immune system is being further weakened with each shot:

> "The numbers in the Denmark study described below are now confirmed by government data from Germany showing that *vaccinated people are 8X more likely to develop Omicron than unvaccinated people.* This is not surprising since a paper from Germany showed the same thing: the more you vaccinate, the worse it gets.
>
> "...*The longer you stay on the vaccine treadmill, the harder to get off in the future and the easier you'll make it for the virus.*
>
> "*In short, we've been lied to about the vaccine.* It is protecting you less and less over time. While you may get a benefit for earlier variants, the benefit for other variants (and likely other diseases) is going to be negative. In short, **you are getting a short term benefit against Delta, but at the expense of a degradation of your overall immunity to everything else.**"[288] (emphasis added)

Dr. Geert Vanden Bossche, DVM, Ph.D. (Virology), is an experienced vaccine developer who has worked with the Bill and Melinda Gates Foundation and the Global Alliance for Vaccine Immunization (GAVI). Since 2020, he has been warning that *these injections would destroy the immune system,* making the vaccinated population vulnerable for every new variant of the disease, not to mention other diseases. He said:

> "Mass vaccination campaigns *during* a pandemic of highly infectious variants fail to control viral transmission. *Instead of contributing to building herd immunity, they dramatically delay natural establishment of herd immunity.* This is why the ongoing universal vaccination campaigns are absolutely detrimental to public and global health...

DESTRUCTIVE IMPACT ON THE NATURAL IMMUNE SYSTEM

"People ... who are not knowledgeable in the fields of immunology, virology, vaccinology and evolutionary biology/epidemiology are, therefore, not a good source for information or advice...

"The mass vaccination hype will undoubtedly enter history as the most reckless experiment in the history of medicine."[289] (emphasis added)

Dr. Deborah Viglione explains that one of the issues causing this is called original antigenic sin. The immune system is being hijacked to only recognize the Wuhan version of the spike protein which no longer exists. Therefore, it is not recognizing the new variants. What is even more concerning is that the immune system may be so tied up looking for the Wuhan virus that it no longer recognizes other viruses such as the flu. The same thing is true of the new Omicron variant (bivalent) shots, as those variants no longer exist, so they are expired vaccines also.

Another problem with the COVID shots is antibody dependent enhancement (ADE). This is an over-reaction of the immune system when a vaccine recipient is actually challenged with the virus. According to Viglione, Thorp and many other doctors, this causes a worse illness and cytokine storm.[290] This was a huge cause of death in the earlier animal trials of coronavirus vaccines. This is also postulated as a cause of the increased hospitalization and death rate that is reported now in the vaccinated versus the unvaccinated population that contracts COVID.

Another potential problem is the possibility of "immune exhaustion." Dr. Ryan Cole explains that this poses a real threat for people who continue to receive boosters.[291] The immune system can become so over-stimulated to a degree that it just "gives up" and is unable to fight other infections and cancer.

How long will these immune system changes last? The earlier version of Moderna's website cited earlier implies that the immune system is only being temporarily evaded just long enough for the lipid nanoparticles to deliver their contents. However, the scientific data is showing that these changes are ongoing and there is huge concern for long-term autoimmune disease. In January 2022, Dr. Ryan Cole stated that "we don't know how long the immune system is suppressed after the shots, and how long these receptors are shut off because those studies aren't done," at least not as of that point in time.[292]

[274] Fohse, F. Konstantin; Gecklin, Buisranur; Overheul, Gijis J. The BNT162b2 mRNA vaccine against SARS-CoV-2 reprograms both adaptive and innate immune responses Research Gate May 2021 doi:10.1101/2021.05.03.21256520 ; also, Seneff S, Nigh G, Kyriakopoulos AM, McCullough PA. Innate immune suppression by SARS-CoV-2 mRNA vaccinations: The role of G-quadruplexes, exosomes, and MicroRNAs. Food Chem Toxicol. 2022 Jun;164:113008. doi: 10.1016/j.fct.2022.113008. Epub 2022 Apr 15. PMID: 35436552; PMCID: PMC9012513. https://www.ncbi.nlm.nih.gov/pmc/articles/PMC9012513/

[275] Karikó K, Muramatsu H, Welsh FA, Ludwig J, Kato H, Akira S, Weissman D. Incorporation of pseudouridine into mRNA yields superior nonimmunogenic vector with increased translational capacity and biological stability. Nov;16(11):1833-40. doi: 10.1038/mt.2008.200. Epub 2008 Sep 16.PMID: 18797453 ; https://pubmed.ncbi.nlm.nih.gov/18797453/

[276] Obeid, Elias; Nanda, Rita; et al. Association of downregulation of toll-like receptor 3 (TLR3) expression with aggressive breast cancer (BC). DOI:10.1200/jco.2013.31.15_suppl.11035 *Journal of Clinical Oncology* 31, no. 15_suppl (May 20, 2013) 11035-11035. https://ascopubs.org/doi/abs/10.1200/jco.2013.31.15_suppl.11035

[277] Torres I, Albert E, et al. B- and T-cell immune responses elicited by the Comirnaty® COVID-19 vaccine in nursing-home residents. Clin Microbiol Infect. 2021 Nov;27(11):1672-1677. doi: 10.1016/j.cmi.2021.06.013. Epub 2021 Jun 24. PMID: 34174397; PMCID: PMC8223011; https://www.sciencegate.app/document/10.1016/j.cmi.2021.06.013; also, Seneff S, Nigh G, Kyriakopoulos AM, McCullough PA. Innate immune suppression by SARS-CoV-2 mRNA vaccinations (cited above)

[278] Liu J, Wang J, et al, Comprehensive investigations revealed consistent pathophysiological alterations after vaccination with COVID-19 vaccines. Cell Discovery (2021) 7:99, https://doi.org/10.1038/s41421-021-00329-3

[279] Torres I, Albert E, et al. B- and T-cell immune responses elicited by the Comirnaty® COVID-19 vaccine in nursing-home residents. Clin Microbiol Infect. 2021 Nov;27(11):1672-1677. doi: 10.1016/j.cmi.2021.06.013. Epub 2021 Jun 24. PMID: 34174397; PMCID: PMC8223011; https://www.sciencegate.app/document/10.1016/j.cmi.2021.06.013;also, Seneff S, Nigh G, Kyriakopoulos AM, McCullough PA. Innate immune suppression by SARS-CoV-2 mRNA vaccinations (cited above)

[280] Singh N, Bharara Singh A. S2 subunit of SARS-nCoV-2 interacts with tumor suppressor protein p53 and BRCA: an in silico study. Transl Oncol. 2020 Oct;13(10):100814. doi: 10.1016/j.tranon.2020.100814. Epub 2020 Jun 30. PMID: 32619819; PMCID: PMC7324311. https://pubmed.ncbi.nlm.nih.gov/32619819/

[281] Liu J, Wang J, et al, Comprehensive investigations revealed consistent pathophysiological alterations after vaccination (cited above)

[282] https://web.archive.org/web/20220114040737/https://www.modernatx.com/mrna-technology/mrna-platform-enabling-drug-discovery-development..

[283] Dr. Ryan Cole. MD interviewed by Dr. Brian Hooker, https://childrenshealthdefense.org/defender/dr-ryan-cole-shots-hooker/ (May 26, 2022)

[284] Dr. Ryan Cole interviewed by Greg Hunter, https://usawatchdog.com/global-cv19-vax-absolute-insanity-dr-ryan-cole/ (June 4, 2022)

[285] Todd Callender interviewed by Reiner Fuellmich, https://www.bitchute.com/video/RS3F9kQAoeCD/ (March 2022)

[286] https://expose-news.com/2022/05/22/your-gov-confirmed-covid-vaccinated-develop-a-id-s-5-months/ (May 22, 2022)

[287] Steve Kirsch, https://stevekirsch.substack.com/p/my-interviews-with-ryan-cole-deb (Aug 13, 2022)

[288] Steve Kirsch "New Studies Show That the COVID Vaccines Damage Your Immune System," https://stevekirsch.substack.com/p/new-study-shows-vaccines-must-be (Dec. 24, 2021). https://stevekirsch.substack.com/p/new-study-from-germany-confirms-higher (Nov. 20, 2021). The German study referred to in Kirsch's article is at https://www.skirsch.com/covid/GermanAnalysis.pdf.

[289] Robin Monotti Gradziadei (Sept 13, 2021) https://nulluslocussinegenio.com/2021/09/13/why-mass-vaccinations-prolong-and-make-epidemics-deadlier-real-vaccine-expert-calls-out-flawed-government-pandemic-strategy/; See also Dr. Geert Vanden Bossche Interview, https://thehighwire.com/videos/a-coming-covid-catastrophe/ (March 11, 2021)

[290] Hagemann K, Riecken K, et al. Natural killer cell-mediated ADCC in SARS-CoV-2-infected individuals and vaccine recipients. Eur J Immunol. 2022 Aug;52(8):1297-1307. doi.10.1002/eji.202149470. Epub 2022 Apr 22. PMID: 35416291; PMCID: PMC9087393; https://onlinelibrary.wiley.com/doi/full/10.1002/eji.202149470; also, Huisman W, Martina BE, Rimmelzwaan GF, Gruters RA, Osterhaus AD. Vaccine-induced enhancement of viral infections. 2009 Jan 22;27(4):505-12. doi: 10.1016/j.vaccine.2008.10.087. Epub 2008 Nov 18. PMID: 19022319. https://pubmed.ncbi.nlm.nih.gov/19022319/

[291] From a presentation by Dr. Ryan Cole, MD, "COVID-19 -Then and Now," at Pensacola, FL (May 19, 2022), as reported by Dr. Deborah Viglione; also, from a presentation by Dr. Ryan Cole, MD, at the Gateway to Freedom conference, Collinsville, IL (Aug. 25-27, 2022), as reported by Dr. Deborah Viglione.

[292] Dr. Ryan Cole, interviewed by Veronika Kyrylenko, https://thenewamerican.com/dr-ryan-cole-covid-vax-damages-your-immune-system/ (Jan. 27, 2022)

Chapter 19
The "Future Framework" for New COVID "Vaccine" Formulations

It is important to be aware of the FDA's new strategy for approving newly reformulated COVID vaccines that was given the green light in late June 2022 – *without any new clinical trials.* Dr. Toby Rogers, Ph.D., an expert on regulatory capture and Big Pharma corruption, addresses the problem that Pfizer and Moderna had been facing:

> "their COVID-19 shots do not stop infection, transmission, hospitalization, nor death from the SARS-CoV-2 virus. Everyone knows this ... Pfizer and Moderna are making about $50 billion a year on these shots and they want that to continue. So they need to reformulate the shots... these shots don't work so it's not clear what it will take to get them to work. This is a problem because reformulated shots mean new clinical trials and new regulatory review by the FDA." [293]

Based on the devastating data surrounding the original COVID shots, the manufacturers might have had a problem surviving that scrutiny. However, because of the strong desire to have newly reformulated shots out by September of 2022, the FDA decided in late June 2022 to follow a new strategy referred to as the "Future Framework." Rogers explains how the Future Framework scheme was proposed to work:

> "all future Covid-19 shots – regardless of the formulation -- will automatically be deemed 'safe and effective' without additional clinical trials, because they are considered 'biologically similar' to existing shots." [294]

Instead, the reformulated COVID shots would be tested on a small number of mice. One article published on August 22, 2022 reports:

"Pfizer noted that it only had efficacy data ... from mice. *In eight mice*, the BA.4/5 bivalent booster generated about a 2.6-fold increase in neutralizing antibody levels against the BA.4/5 subvariants compared with the companies' current booster. The companies presented that mouse data to the FDA in June."[295]

There is the data – 8 mice. And that is only *efficacy* data, *not safety* data. There was no safety data. Apparently, according Rogers, the plan is to watch for safety signals *after* the products are released into the marketplace, "using a safety system no one has ever heard of while ignoring the system that has existed for 32 years that is showing a massive safety signal right now."[296] Moreover, what little efficacy data there was, it was only short-term. We know from earlier efficacy data in humans that it was short-lived and ultimately disastrous. *Is there any reason to expect these new formulations would be any different, given how quickly mutations occur?*

Toby Rogers watched the FDA meeting in late June at which the decision was made to go ahead with this new approach. He stated that he may have been the only one who noticed the note in the bottom corner of a presentation slide that the "immunogenicity data" was based on the 8 mice. The same organization that published the above August 22 report also had an email confirmation from Pfizer that "it hadn't collected any new preclinical efficacy data since then." John Moore, a New York immunologist, expressed his opinion: "For the FDA to rely on mouse data is just bizarre ... Mouse data are not going to be predictive in any way of what you would see in humans."[297] Dr. Peter McCullough agrees, and describes the FDA's new approach as "wide open malfeasance and corruption."[298]

Pfizer/BioNTech announced on August 22, 2022, that they had just submitted their new drug application to the FDA, for EUA of its new bivalent Omicron BA.4/BA.5 vaccine under this new framework.[299] The new formulation "contains mRNA encoding the original SARS-CoV-2 spike protein," as well as the "spike protein of the Omicron CA.4/BA.5 variant." *Why would they include encoding for the original Wuhan strain since that was already long past?* Those who support the expedited process justify it on the basis of their belief that the original COVID vaccines are safe and effective, and that there is no time to wait for human clinical trials.[300] The latter point actually shows why a vaccine was never an appropriate intervention in the first place, as discussed in Part 1. It also is a clear rejection of the "rule" often voiced by Dr. Peter McCullough that it is always about *safety first* – "safety, safety, safety."

Rogers also commented that before his fight to try to stop the FDA from approving these shots, "the FDA pretended to be a regulatory agency." However, what became clear to him by late June, when the FDA decided to start implementing the Future Framework, was the following:

> "the FDA absolutely does not care about science nor health. Furthermore we discovered that the FDA has been laundering Moderna and Pfizer's data for them throughout the Emergency Use Authorization process. And now the FDA is abandoning clinical trials altogether in connection with Covid-19 shots. What an extraordinary admission of failure on their part. We now know that the FDA is NOT a regulatory agency. The FDA is the data laundering branch of the Pharma cartel." [301]

Is it perhaps way past time to re-visit the assumptions that a vaccine is even necessary in the first place, and that no therapeutic treatments are available? *Is it not time to wake up to the reality that the regulatory agencies have been captured by Big Pharma, and what that means for public health as well as the future of the entire health care system?*

The more the medical industrial complex keeps pushing COVID boosters, the more everyone should be asking *why*, and *who is really benefitting* from these endless shots. *Doctors, do you believe you can honestly advise your patients that any of the reformulated COVID shots are safe and effective without any clinical trials? If so, are you prepared to defend that position with solid data from sources that have no conflicts of interest?*

In turning now to look at many of the serious irregularities and manipulations that have characterized the regulatory process in connection with the COVID shots, consider how the "Future Framework" strategy puts Big Pharma profits ahead of public health. Make a mental checklist of the many kinds of corrupt practices that the manufacturers will be able to get away with much more easily now without having to do any clinical trials.

---

[293] Toby Rogers, PhD, https://brownstone.org/articles/the-fdas-future-framework-for-covid-vaccines-is-reckless-plan/ (June 22, 2022)

[294] Id.

[295] Beth Mole, https://arstechnica.com/science/2022/08/with-data-in-mice-pfizer-asks-fda-to-authorize-its-fall-ba-4-5-booster-shot/ (Aug. 22, 2022)

[296] Toby Rogers, https://tobyrogers.substack.com/p/the-end-of-covid-19-vaccine-safety (June 29, 2022)

[297] Rob Stein, https://www.nprillinois.org/2022-08-18/whats-behind-the-fdas-controversial-strategy-for-evaluating-new-covid-boosters (Aug. 18, 2022)

[298] Dr. Peter McCullough interviewed by Nadera Lopez-Garrity, https://childrenshealthdefense.org/video-post/new-generation-of-covid-19-shots-what-you-must-know-with-dr-peter-mccullough/ (Sept. 5, 2022)

[299] https://www.pfizer.com/news/press-release/press-release-detail/pfizer-and-biontech-submit-application-us-fda-emergency-use (Aug. 22, 2022)

[300] Rob Stein, https://www.nprillinois.org/2022-08-18/whats-behind-the-fdas-controversial-strategy-for-evaluating-new-covid-boosters (Aug. 18, 2022)

[301] Toby Rogers, https://tobyrogers.substack.com/p/the-end-of-covid-19-vaccine-safety (June 29, 2022)

Chapter 20
Pfizer Documents Show Other Irregularities in Manufacturing, Reporting and Clinical Trials

Many other Pfizer documents have been released that reveal various safety-related concerns as well as issues showing lack of disclosure or misrepresentations of important information. For example, an article in *TrialSiteNews* reported as early as May 2021 that regulatory documents show that Pfizer either did not conduct certain routine testing prior to launching the COVID vaccines, or they did not do them properly.[302] EMA documents stated: "'No traditional pharmacokinetic or biodistribution studies have been performed with the vaccine candidate BNT162b2.'" Upon reviewing EMA's evaluation, Dr. Robert Malone "was particularly surprised that the dossier of regulatory documents indicates allowance for use in humans based on non-GLP PK and Tox studies relying on formulations which are significantly different from the final vaccine," That same article also reported that "Pfizer did not follow industry-standard quality management practices during preclinical toxicology studies during vaccines, as key studies did not meet good laboratory practice (GLP). The full panel of industry-standard reproductive toxicity and genotoxicity studies were apparently also not performed."

Pre-EUA Document Showing Knowledge of Potential Issues. A document entitled "FDA Safety Surveillance of COVID-19 Vaccines DRAFT Working List of possible adverse event outcomes"[303] was presented by the FDA on October 22, 2020 at a committee presentation, several weeks *before* FDA's grants of Emergency Use Authorization. That document listed several health risks that the FDA had already known about and identified that were associated with animal studies *before* issuing its EUA for the COVID shots. Among the many risks listed on page 16 of that presentation are death, myocarditis/pericarditis, stroke, autoimmune disease, adverse pregnancy and birth outcomes, Guillain-Barre, anaphylaxis, convulsions/seizures, thrombocytopenia, vaccine enhanced disease and more. *If health care providers and the general public had been aware of this information, how do you think it would have affected their decision to recommend, administer or receive the shots?*

Documents Show Misrepresentations of Serious Adverse Event Classifications. An article in *The Defender* dated June 21, 2022, focused on 80,000 pages of Pfizer documents released on June 1 which included a large number of case reports.[304] The documents "reveal a trend of classifying almost all adverse events – and in particular severe adverse events (SAEs) – as being 'not related' to the vaccine." Among other things, these events included acute respiratory failure, cardiac arrest, brain abscess, adrenal carcinoma and chronic myeloid leukemia. The article claims "This isn't believable. It's completely unrealistic, especially when serious events occur in multiple participants." "Many participants also dropped out or were excluded from the trial due to serious side effects involving the heart, cardiovascular system, cancer, stroke, hemorrhage and neurological impacts." Most Level 3 adverse events were also declared to be unrelated to the shot. One document had a table labelled "Potential side effects of BNT162b2" which shows myocarditis as a "rare" potential side effect, but defined "rare" as affecting "between 1 in 1,000 and 1 in 10,000 people."[305] *Do you consider that "rare"?*

The case of Maddie de Garay is a classic example of Pfizer's dismissal of certain adverse reactions as being serious. Maddie was a healthy 12-year-old when she enrolled in the 12 to 15-year-old Pfizer clinical trials. According to a letter from her attorneys to government officials,[306] within 24 hours of Maddie's second dose, she suffered "crippling, scream-inducing pain" that landed her in the ER. She had severe chest and abdominal pains that she said felt like "[her] heart was being ripped out through [her] neck." She was hospitalized three times over the next few months. She has been confined to a wheelchair, has to be tube fed and suffers many other life-changing symptoms: "gastroparesis, erratic blood pressure, erratic heart rate, memory loss, brain fog, dizziness, fainting, seizures, verbal tics, motor tics, loss of feeling from her waist through her toes, muscle weakness, drastic and adverse changes in her vision, urinary retention, loss of bladder control, and the start of and severely irregular menstrual cycles." ***How did Pfizer report this in their clinical trial documents to the FDA?*** "Functional abdominal pain."

What is equally reprehensible is that doctors who examined Maddie afterwards made a diagnosis of "functional neurological syndrome." They concluded that Maddie's problems were all in her head and not a vaccine injury, even though her symptoms started within 24 hours of her second dose, and she had previously been a healthy child. In an August 2022 interview, Maddie's parents shared how they felt "abandoned" and "left high and dry" as they desperately tried to get help for Maddie.[307] ***Imagine if that had happened to your child.***

Serious Issues Revealed in Leaked Emails. In 2020, a cybersecurity breach resulted in the leak of many emails and other documents revealing interactions between the European Medicines Agency (EMA – Europe's "FDA") and Pfizer in November 2020. That was just a few weeks before Pfizer was granted its EUA from the FDA and the regulators in the UK and Europe granted their corresponding authorizations. Several major issues were revealed.

One of the EMA's major objections-was the integrity of the mRNA, as reflected in wide variation between batches.[308] That variation is also reflected in the Paardekooper/Team Enigma research findings of huge inconsistencies across batches, as discussed below, but their research was based on the number of serious adverse events associated with each particular batch *after the rollout, not on pre-rollout* findings.

This issue from a pre-EUA and pre-rollout perspective was the subject of review by Alexandra "Sasha" Latypova, a former pharmaceutical and biotech industry executive who "spent 25 years in pharmaceutical research and development working with more than 60 companies worldwide to submit data to the FDA on hundreds of clinical trials."[309] She was asked to give a witness statement about this issue, based on the leaked documents from the EMA.[310]

In addition to noting the "excessive variations" in the safety profiles between batches, she attests to the following in her affidavit:

1. "The modified RNA (mRNA) which is the active substance of Pfizer's vaccine BNT162b2 is allowed to vary in its integrity by up to 50% in the finished product.

2. "Product impurities in the form of truncated mRNA, untranslated DNA and other unknown nucleic acid constructs have been allowed in the finished product in unspecified quantities."

She also noted that these impurities were found only several days before it gained authorization to be released to the public. Pfizer and BioNTech had repeatedly stated that efficacy of their product was dependent on the "quantity of sufficiently intact mRNA" and "even a minor degradation" could have a "severe" effect on performance. Furthermore, she noted changes that were made in the manufacturing process to scale up:

"[they] were performed without re-validation of the manufacturing process or re-running the preclinical and clinical studies to confirm comparability on safety and efficacy characteristics of the product. Importantly, these changes resulted in a substantial drop in the integrity of key active ingredient – mRNA … in each manufactured batch. This was identified by the regulatory reviewers at EMA and FDA, and EMA specifically recorded this as a Major Objection #2, i.e. a regulatory flag that required a resolution prior to the product approval."

That issue was discussed at a meeting between EMA and Pfizer on November 26, 2020 as evidenced in one of the documents Latypova reviewed. She says that they apparently resolved this objection "by arbitrarily lowering the acceptance criteria for %mRNA integrity." The UK gave its authorization on December 2, the FDA on December 11 and the EMA on December 21.[311] Her affidavit also says:

"An extremely wide variation of the integrity of the active substance in bulk material (batch) of the product and abundant presence of uncharacterized impurities means that batches of different formulation … are being produced. This variation is further amplified when the bulk material is filled in small quantities into vials. Each batch of Pfizer product contains approximately 300,000 vials…"

Latypova also noted that: "Both the regulators and Pfizer to date have not disclosed the acceptable ranges for the key ingredients of the vaccine product, neither in bulk product nor in a vial (as dispensed), and claim 'commercial secrets' that prevent them from doing so." Latypova's third finding expresses other serious concerns:

3. "As a result of the reckless widening of quality acceptance criteria for the integrity of active ingredient in manufacturing batches, there is a great variation in resulting formulations of final product as dispensed in vials. Furthermore, the contents of the vials are cut by hand into multiple doses by untrained and unsupervised vaccinators who are working outside of the Good Manufacturing Practice compliance."

Who are the people doing that task, and is such "hand-cutting" a common practice in the production of other pharmaceuticals? She concluded:

"the evidence presented in my statement shows that Pfizer's manufacturing quality acceptance criteria permit for an extremely large variation of the key ingredient (up to 50%) and allow for a substantial presence of uncharacterized impurities. This can be deemed as product adulteration..."

Other analyses of the EMA documents on this issue of mRNA integrity and the inconsistency between batches reveal a lack of serious concern by at least some regulators. An article by investigative journalist Sonia Elijah in *TrialSiteNews.com*[312] revealed the following information. A November 24, 2020 email from Veronika Jekerle, PhD, Head of EMA's Office of Pharmaceutical Quality Office, states that most of the member states shared "a number of [remaining] major concerns that impact the benefit/risk of the vaccine (efficacy/safety) most notably the comparability issue around the % mRNA integrity." Jekerle sent another email on November 24 stating that "FDA/HC [Health Canada]/EMA agreed that alignment on specifications % mRNA integrity are key in order **to avoid that one regions [*sic*} gets all the suboptimal material**..." (emphasis added)

However, around the same time, Elijah reports, Marco Cavaleri, then the EMA's Head of Biological Health Threats and Vaccines Strategy, stated in an email that "the issue on the mRNA content not perceived as major." He also stated: "unclear if GCP [Good Clinical Practise] inspections ever done... but no major interest from FDA." Sonia Elijah then referenced one of her own previous articles stating that the FDA had inspected only 1% of Pfizer's trial sites. *It appears that the FDA was not very concerned about the manufacturers' compliance with safety standards and practices for this novel experimental drug.*

Whistleblower Report of Clinical Trial Irregularities. Major problems with Pfizer's clinical trials that affected the quality of the trial data, and the company's knowledge of those problems, were reported by whistleblower Brook Jackson. Jackson served briefly as a regional manager for Ventavia, one of Pfizer's clinical trial contractors during Phase 3 of its COVID-19 vaccine trials. She had over 15 years of experience in clinical research coordination and management as of September 2020 when she went to work for Ventavia. She was responsible for overseeing three trial sites in Texas involving over 1,000 participants. Jackson told *The BMJ*[313] that during her work with Ventavia, among other unacceptable actions she witnessed:

> "the company falsified data, unblinded patients, employed inadequately trained vaccinators, and was slow to follow up on adverse events reported in Pfizer's pivotal phase III trial. Staff who conducted quality control checks were overwhelmed by the volume of problems they were finding."

Though she repeatedly reported the problems to her superiors, they did nothing. In a meeting she had with two company directors, the *BMJ* article reports that "a Ventavia executive can be heard explaining that the company wasn't able to quantify the types and number of errors they were finding when examining the trial paperwork for quality control." One executive said: "In my mind, it's something new every day...We know that it's significant." The next morning, September 25, 2020, Jackson contacted the FDA by phone, warning about unsound practices she experienced at Ventavia. She then sent the FDA an email explaining her concerns. That afternoon Jackson was fired.

After Jackson left Ventavia, several others either left or were also fired, including one of the Ventavia officials in the meeting referred to above. He told Jackson: "everything that you complained about was spot on." Another former employee commented to the *BMJ* about the data Ventavia generated for Pfizer, saying: "'I don't think it was good clean data... It's a crazy mess.'" Before Jackson left, she gathered evidence of the problems. She has since filed a lawsuit against Ventavia, Pfizer and another entity for violations of the False Claims Act. [314]

---

[302] https://www.trialsitenews.com/a/did-pfizer-fail-to-perform-industry-standard-animal-testing-prior-to-initiation-of-mrna-clinical-trials (May 28, 2021)

[303] https://www.fda.gov/media/143557/download

[304] Michael Nevradakis, Ph.D., "Pfizer Classified Almost All Adverse Events During COVID Vaccine Trials 'Not related to shots,' https://childrenshealthdefense.org/defender/pfizer-covid-vaccine-trials-adverse-events-shots-fda-eua-documents/ (June 21, 2022)

[305] Daniel Horowitz, https://www.conservativereview.com/horowitz-what-did-pfizer-know-and-when-3-important-findings-from-recent-document-releases-2657115084.html (April 7, 2022)

[306] Letter from attorneys Aaron Siri and Elizabeth A. Brehm, Oct. 22, 2021, to Xavier Becerra (HHS Secretary), Dr. Rochelle Walensky (CDC Director), Dr Janet Woodcock (Interim FDA Commissioner), Dr. Peter Marks and Dr. Tom Shimabukuro (CDC COVID-19 Vaccine Task Force); https://www.sirillp.com/wp-content/uploads/2021/10/Letter-to-Federal-Health-Agencies-Regarding-Maddie-and-Clinical-Trials-for-Children.pdf

[307] Segment of Maddie de Garay's parents' interview with Highwire host Del Bigtree (Aug. 2022) in the documentary, *Rigged*, https://thehighwire.com/videos/rigged-maddies-story/

[308] Sasha Latypova, https://www.trialsitenews.com/a/my-affidavit-on-different-formulations-in-pfizer-vaccine-lots-1b9e4ee9 (June 30, 2022)

[309] Megan Redshaw, https://childrenshealthdefense.org/defender/fda-moderna-bypass-covid-vaccine-safety-standards-documents/ (July 12, 2022)

[310] Sasha Latypova, https://www.trialsitenews.com/a/my-affidavit-on-different-formulations-in-pfizer-vaccine-lots-1b9e4ee9 (June 30, 2022)

[311] Sonia Elijah, https://www.trialsitenews.com/a/what-the-leaked-ema-emails-docs-reveal-major-concerns-with-pfizer-c-19-vaccine-batch-integrity-and-the-race-to-authorise-cdda0ba2 (June 20, 2022)

[312] Id.

[313] Thacker P D. COVID-19: Researcher blows the whistle on data integrity issues in Pfizer's vaccine trial. *BMJ* 2021; 375 :n2635 doi:10.1136/bmj.n2635; https://www.bmj.com/content/375/bmj.n2635

[314] https://www.documentcloud.org/documents/21206071-brook-jackson-lawsuit

Chapter 21
Moderna's Improprieties

Moderna has its share of improprieties as well. An August 2021 article[315] reported that a whistleblower from a company that works with Moderna in handling its adverse reaction reports had made a screenshot of an internal company document. It showed that *Moderna had received 300,000 reports of adverse reactions within a 3-month period.* Moderna is legally required to submit all such reports to VAERS, but that figure was said to "dwarf" the number showing in VAERS for any 3-month period up to that point. **Why were these not reported to VAERS? How many more reports does Moderna need before it detects a warning signal?**

Even worse are allegations from Sasha Latypova, the former pharmaceutical and biotech industry executive quoted above. In an article entitled "FDA Colluded with Moderna to Bypass COVID Vaccine Safety Standards, Documents, Reveal," in *The Defender* published by Children's Health Defense, Latypova reveals results of her review of 699 pages from the HHS of "studies and test results 'supposedly used by the FDA to clear Moderna's mRNA platform-based-mRNA 1273, or Spikevax.'"[316] In Latypova's opinion, the documents suggest that the FDA and Moderna "colluded to bypass regulatory and scientific standards used to ensure products are safe." She said:

> "It is evident that the FDA and NIH [National Institutes of Health] colluded with Moderna to subvert the regulatory and scientific standards of drug safety testing...
>
> "They accepted fraudulent test designs, substitutions of test articles, glaring omissions and whitewashing of serious signs of health damage by the product, then lied to the public on behalf of the manufacturers."

In an earlier op-ed in *TrialSiteNews*,[317] she summarized her findings as follows:

1. "Moderna's nonclinical summary contains mostly irrelevant materials.
2. Moderna claims that the active substance mRNAs of Spikevax does not need to be studied for toxicity and can be replaced with any other mRNA without further testing.
3. Moderna's nonclinical program consisted of studies of other unapproved mRNAs and only one non-GLP toxicology study of mRNA-1273 (active substance of SPIKEVAX).
4. There are two separate Investigational New Drug numbers for mRNA-1273: one held by Moderna, the other – by DMID (NIH), representing a serious conflict of interest.
5. The vaccine-induced antibody-enhanced disease was identified as a serious risk and was not excluded by Moderna due to absence of positive control and unvalidated methods used.
6. FDA and Moderna lied about reproductive toxicology studies in public disclosures and product labeling."

In elaborating on the first finding, she said that about "80% of materials included in the package are for other mRNA products unrelated to Sars-Cov-2 or covid illness. The entire package is haphazardly organized, possibly on purpose, to make it harder to read and interpret." She also stated:

> "Curiously, the approved Moderna SPIKEVAX label does not contain any information regarding the concentration of the product supplied in the vials. [footnote deleted]
>
> "Finally, all documents are poorly and often incompetently written. There are numerous hypothetical statements unsupported by any data, proposed theories, admissions of using unvalidated assays, and repetitive paragraphs throughout. Quite shockingly, this represents the entire safety toxicology assessment for an extremely novel product that has gotten injected into millions of arms worldwide."

With regard to her second finding above, she analogized to two trucks, one carrying food and one carrying explosives, with the companies taking the position that the two are the same thing. In other words, she says: "Ignore the cargo, focus on the vehicle. The claim is preposterous." This appears to be the same reasoning behind the FDA's decision in late June 2022 to follow the "Future Framework" strategy for new formulations of the COVID "vaccines," discussed earlier. That new approach allows the manufacturers to gain approval or authorization of their "reformulated" products *without any new clinical trials*.[318] However, what Latypova discusses next raises serious questions about the validity and wisdom of the Future Framework as applied to COVID vaccines.

Latypova also presents the manufacturers' claim: "If mRNA works once, it will work many times." But she also noted that the European regulatory reviewers of Pfizer's mRNA product stated that it was the "modified mRNA" that was the new chemical entity, not just the lipid envelope. She also stated that "All new chemical entities must undergo rigorous safety testing before they are approved as medicinal products in the United States, Europe and the rest of the world.'" On the basis of the documents she had seen so far, Latypova concluded:

> "the manufacturer's claim is not supported by any real data, no studies are cited showing that all toxicity of the product resides with the lipid envelope and none with the 'payload' of the type and sequence of mRNA delivered to various tissues and organs."

Latypova also noted that the FDA had been providing guidance documents for cellular and gene therapies since 1998, so there already existed a large body of information about testing requirements for this class of product prior to the COVID vaccines.

> "These materials documented many serious risks, including death, potential to promote cancer, uncontrollable expression of proteins, genotoxicity, reproductive harm, and potential for transmission through 'shedding,' among many others. The manufacturers and regulators both were expected to anticipate these risks and design testing programs to exclude or fully characterize them."

She also said that "Pharmacokinetics (Biodistribution) were not studied with the SPIKEVAX mRNA-1273." Also: "No metabolism, excretion, pharmacokinetic drug interactions, or any other pharmacokinetic studies for mRNA-1273 were conducted. There were no safety pharmacology assessments for any organ classes such as cardiovascular, CNS, liver, spleen, etc."

With regard to Latypova's 5th finding, she notes that Moderna had never brought an approved drug to market before. She pointed out the company's history of many failed products: "Notably, its mRNA-based vaccines were associated with the antibody-dependent enhancement phenomenon." Yet, she says, Moderna apparently "dismissed this extremely significant risk without a proper study design." There is more information in that same *TrialSiteNews* article about Latypova's other findings from the Moderna documents. But the above should be more than enough to raise serious concerns about the basis on which Moderna's Spikevax mRNA-1273 product cleared the FDA's review.

---

[315] Alex Berenson, "Some Actual news about Moderna adverse event reports," https://alexberenson.substack.com/p/some-actual-news (Aug. 6, 2021)

[316] Megan Redshaw, https://childrenshealthdefense.org/defender/fda-moderna-bypass-covid-vaccine-safety-standards-documents/ (July 12, 2022)

[317] Sasha Latypova, https://www.trialsitenews.com/a/modernas-non-clinical-summary-for-spikevax-evidence-of-scientific-and-regulatory-fraud-fd53b4f7#_ftn4 (July 6, 2022)

[318] Mary Villareal, https://www.chemicalviolence.com/2022-07-14-fda-future-framework-allows-bypass-vaccine-testing.html (July 14, 2022)

Chapter 22
Problems with the Johnson & Johnson COVID Shots

Although the vast bulk of evidence in this book has focused on the Pfizer and Moderna vaccines, since theirs have been the most widely administered in the U.S., other COVID vaccine manufacturers and their COVID products present similar issues and have been prone to various problems. First, it should be noted that although other COVID vaccines use a different delivery system than the mRNA technology used by Pfizer and Moderna, they also are injecting genetic materials.[319] Therefore, those who received COVID vaccines made by other companies should not think that they are safe from all of the problems reported with respect to the mRNA shots.

Johnson & Johnson received its EUA on February 27, 2021. Only six weeks later, on April 13, the FDA and CDC recommended a pause in its administration "to investigate six reported cases of TTS [thrombosis with thrombocytopenia syndrome], and to help ensure that health care providers were made aware of the potential for TTS…"[320] It is commendable that they paused to investigate only six cases of one condition, but the huge question that raises is: *why was J & J singled out for 6 cases of TTS while reports of thousands of deaths and many more thousands of other serious conditions following Pfizer's and Moderna's COVID vaccines were apparently ignored and their vaccines were not paused in the U.S.?* From an attorney's perspective, that looks extremely suspicious. On April 23, following what it called "a thorough safety investigation," according to the FDA website, the FDA and CDC lifted the pause, even though 7 more cases of TTS had been reported by then, out of about 8 million doses. They asserted that the benefits still outweighed the risks for those 18 and older.

A couple months later, in July 2021, the J & J shot was "dealt another blow" when about 100 cases of the rare autoimmune disorder, Guillain-Barre syndrome (GBS) were reported, out of 12.5 million doses. Of those,

95 were serious, and one died.[321] Interestingly, as pointed out earlier, it was several cases of that disorder which led to the complete stoppage of the 1976 swine flu vaccine campaign, which the CDC at that time said was necessary based only on *"the possibility of an association of GBS with the vaccine, however small."*[322] The FDA then put a warning on the J & J product, suggesting there was an increased risk of GBS *up to 42 days after vaccination.* As the data reported earlier in Parts 1 and 2 of this book show, there have been exponentially more reports of blood clotting, Guillain-Barre and many other serious problems, *including death,* following Pfizer and Moderna injections. **Why were they not subjected to the same scrutiny as J & J?**

In its May 5, 2022 announcement to limit the use of the J&J vaccine to certain persons, the director of FDA's Center for Biologics Evaluation and Research stated that their action "demonstrates the robustness of our safety surveillance systems and our commitment to ensuring that science and data guide our decisions." An updated analysis on TTS, also reported in the FDA's May 5, 2022 announcement, shows that there was a total of 60 confirmed TTS cases reported to VAERS through March 18, 2022, including 9 cases resulting in death.

If they are truly committed to letting science and data guide their decisions, why has there been no pause of either Pfizer's or Moderna's COVID vaccines? What should we make of these glaring inconsistencies in the FDA's treatment of the various COVID vaccine manufacturers? It should also be noted that they acknowledged the possibility of a causal link between GBS and the vaccine even if symptoms might not show up for 42 days. *However, they have been very quick to conclude there was no causal link between the vaccines and other serious symptoms, including deaths, that have occurred within only hours, days or even a few weeks of injection.* **Why is that?**

J&J has been plagued by serious manufacturing problems as well. A House of Representatives subcommittee did an investigation of the problems at the Emergent BioSolutions plant that was producing both the J&J and AstraZeneca COVID vaccines. It presented its findings and a more detailed history of the manufacturing problems in a May 2022 Staff Report.[323] That report reveals poor quality control and a variety of GMP (Good Manufacturing Practices) compliance failures, as well as high turnover among its staff and inadequate training and experience of its employees. It also revealed a general lack of capabilities to handle this anticipated production. In early 2021, employees at the plant accidentally cross-contaminated up to about 15 million doses of the J & J vaccine with an ingredient from the AstraZeneca vaccine, which was being produced at the same plant.[324] The FDA shut the plant down in April 2021, but allowed it to resume production in August 2021, even though the FDA had not made an on-site inspection at the plant since July 2021, according to the May 2022 Staff Report. However, the report also stated that the FDA "had not cleared" any J & J batches since production resumed in August 2021. *But why would it have allowed production to resume without an on-site inspection?*

The report also revealed that a total of about 400 million doses had to be terminated or thrown out due to various problems. The company's CEO "blamed the factory's problems on the complexity of scaling up production quickly on two different vaccines."[325] The plant stopped manufacturing in February 2022. In August 2022, it was reported that about 135 million more doses of J & J's vaccines (that had been manufactured before the shutdown) would have to be destroyed due to quality problems,[326] but that might also have had to do with their expiration date.

J & J's COVID vaccine was also being produced in a plant in the Netherlands. However, in February 2022 it was reported that in late 2021, J & J had temporarily shut down that plant, reportedly because it was working on another experimental vaccine unrelated to COVID. J & J said it had millions of doses in its inventory to fulfill its orders.[327] A spokesperson refused to deny or confirm the temporary shutdown. *Why would they refuse to do that? What is going on with J & J?* Needless to say, these problems do not instill confidence.

---

[319] Dr. Peter Breggin, MD and Ginger Ross Breggin, *COVID-19 and the Global Predators: We are the Prey* (2021), pp. 175-178

[320] https://www.fda.gov/news-events/press-announcements/coronavirus-covid-19-update-fda-limits-use-janssen-covid-19-vaccine-certain-individuals (May 5, 2022)

[321] Judy George, https://www.medpagetoday.com/infectiousdisease/covid19vaccine/93537 (July 12, 2021, updated July 13, 2021)

[322] https://www.cdc.gov/vaccinesafety/concerns/concerns-history.html (last accessed May 6, 2022)

[323] Staff Report, Select Subcommittee on the Coronavirus Crisis, Committee on Oversight and Reform, "The Coronavirus Vaccine Manufacturing Failures of Emergent Biosolutions." https://coronavirus.house.gov/sites/democrats.coronavirus.house.gov/files/Coronavirus%20Vaccine%20Manufacturing%20Failures%20of%20Emergent%20BioSolutions.pdf (May 2022)

[324] Sharon Lafraniere and Noah Weiland, https://www.nytimes.com/2021/03/31/world/johnson-and-johnson-vaccine-mixup.html (March 31, 2021)

[325] https://apnews.com/article/covid-business-health-carolyn-maloney-congress-6e649ca8b24fe238cb76ff49284fd59b (May 10, 2022)

[326] https://www.local10.com/news/politics/2022/08/11/jj-covid-vaccine-factory-forced-to-trash-even-more-doses/ (Aug. 11, 2022)

[327] Jake Epstein, https://www.businessinsider.com/johnson-and-johnson-to-shut-down-coronavirus-vaccine-production-report-2022-2 (Feb. 8, 2022).

Chapter 23
Other Evidence That Raises Concerns About Safety

Huge Differences in Numbers of Adverse Events From Different Batches

The issue of the large variation of the mRNA prior to the EUA being granted was discussed above in the affidavit of Sasha Latypova in the section about revelations in the Pfizer documents. One of the points she also referred to were other researchers' findings of huge differences in the numbers of reported adverse events, including deaths, between different batches from the same manufacturer after the vaccines were rolled out, at least in the early batches. Normally the number of adverse events reported is fairly consistent from batch to batch from any given manufacturer. However, this was not the case with the COVID vaccines, according to an analysis done by a researcher from the UK named Craig Paardekooper that was confirmed by an international group called Team Enigma.[328] Their research used the VAERS data to analyze the number of deaths and other adverse reactions reported after COVID-19 vaccinations according to lot numbers. [329]

The data for the COVID-19 vaccines showed huge spikes for many of the lots. According to Sasha Latypova, also a member of Team Enigma, it was initially thought that about 90% of adverse events were coming from only 5% of the lots, based on raw VAERS data at the end of 2021.[330] However, after further research and the Team's discovery of data manipulation by the CDC, the exact percentage of lots responsible for almost all of the adverse event reports cannot be determined. Nevertheless, Latypova says, it is still fair to say that only a small percentage of lots had a very high proportion of adverse event and death reports, while other lots appeared to have many fewer reports in VAERS. After reviewing the initial reports of this huge discrepancy, former Pfizer V.P. and scientist Dr. Michael Yeadon said: "This information about different safety profiles of different 'lots' is completely without precedent."[331] Although the revised percentage may be higher than when he made that statement, his statement most likely still holds true because the relative size of the discrepancy still exits. He concluded that this could only be deliberate because drug manufacturers know how to produce consistent products. Yeadon also called for an immediate stop to these shots, suggesting that a failure to do so is a test of the integrity of the manufacturers and the regulators. People can check the safety profile of their doses at www.HowBadIsMyBatch.com.

The lack of a consistent safety profile across all batches from the same manufacturer is clear. Therefore, the issue is: *what caused such a large discrepancy between batches? Was it due to degradation of the vaccines resulting from the labile nature of the contents in multi-dose vials, or vials having multiple doses administered at different times where the vials were taken in and out of the required very low temperature storage?* Consider whether the discrepancies in adverse reactions might have been due more to what Latypova reported above, about the "extremely wide variation of the integrity of the active substance in bulk material (batch) of the product and abundant presence of uncharacterized impurities [which] means that batches of different formulation … are being produced."

Consider also what Latypova reported about the contents of the vials being "cut by hand into multiple doses by untrained and unsupervised vaccinators who are working outside of the Good Manufacturing Practice compliance." Based on what we know about the manufacturers' conduct in many other aspects of the whole process – many irregularities and improprieties, misrepresentations, lack of compliance, ignoring safety signals, etc. – *is it possible that they might have done something or added something in the preparation or mixing stage that could account for the large numbers of reported AEs and deaths and the large discrepancies between batches?*

To the extent that the excessive variation in the number of AEs between batches is a result of different formulations of the product, has that problem identified by the regulatory agencies been resolved yet? If not, or if we simply do not know, can anyone still say that the vaccines are safe?

Additional Information from Dr. Michael Yeadon

Dr. Michael Yeadon has provided a great deal more key information on the safety issue.[332] Besides having worked for Pfizer, he worked for 32 years in the biopharmaceutical industry years as a biologist, and in immunology, toxicology, and biochemistry, and 10 years in biotech. Therefore, he understands how things are done in the drug industry. He believes the COVID "vaccines" are "very bad products ... a fake vaccine, badly developed, badly designed...These ["vaccines"] are what I would call toxic by design."

He explained that you cannot just scale up the same process for manufacturing billions of doses as you used to make just tens of thousands of doses for clinical trials. He said it's a "very, very complicated process" that requires you "to start again and develop an industrial scale process." He stated:

> "the idea that they got all those processes set up, stabilized, characterized, inspected, agreed by the regulators *is for the birds*. They did not do these things because it's not possible to do them in under a small number of years, probably at least 5 years. What they claim to have done, consistent manufacture, is impossible, and the regulators know it is impossible."

Yeadon had read the same leaked regulatory interactions between the European Medicines Agency (EMA) and Pfizer that Sasha Latypova based her analysis on. While evaluating Pfizer's EUA application, the technical assessors had 7 major objections. Yeadon said the documents showed that "[Pfizer] did not have control of the processes giving rise to consistent pure material. And they didn't have control of what happened to it."

To put this in context, Yeadon's experience at Pfizer was *that if there was even ONE major objection* in the process, *"heads would roll* because it meant you would not have had a dialogue with the regulators so as to understand what was required by them." He said there is no way 7 major objections could have been resolved in only the few weeks' time before they were conveyed to Pfizer by the EMA and when its conditional marketing authorization was given. That was also the conclusion of several colleagues he had spoken to about this. Therefore, in his opinion:

> "So what they have issued and rolled out ...are materials which from batch to batch, vial to vial ... they've got no idea what you're actually getting ... the average should be pretty much the same, and yet they're so different ... it's not the same stuff in each...of the lots. So I would say it's a criminal manufacture, the authorization by the European Medicines Agency and subsequently other global regulators. I think there's criminal level of collusion and fraud to sign off these packages as suitable when absolutely...

it's impossible that they were… And none of the normal processes have been followed. And as a result, it ended up with products that are rushed, dangerous, … intrinsically poor and variable quality. And then the moves to inject the population, including mostly people who are not at any risk from the virus. I hope it will tell you, this whole thing is a fraud, the entire thing is a fraud."

Even before emergency authorization, he and others had tried bringing these matters to the attention of the regulators and the media. Their efforts were ignored. *That, he says, "tells you everything you need to know that it wasn't about public health…"* He warned: "we must stay hypervigilant for what else might be coming." In other words, if the people pushing "vaccines" are not stopped, expect additional outbreaks of something for which they will try to push even more injections for mass distribution. Indeed, what he said is already happening.

Observations from a Pfizer Whistleblower (former employee)

In an interview with Brannon Howse, a Pfizer whistleblower who is now a former employee provided information that corroborates Yeadon's statements as well as additional issues.[333] She said that *Pfizer employees themselves are concerned about what they are seeing in the process of manufacturing. If they are concerned, shouldn't we be also?* The whistleblower said that she and other employees felt very uncomfortable about how these vaccines were being rushed through the process. She had been a manufacturing quality auditor and said that normally, there are *always* stoppages along the way – such as for getting signatures before moving on to the next stage, or hold backs (in the quality control process). She said the process *never* goes totally smoothly and seamlessly, *except in the case of these vaccines*. She said "it's like a seamless process, just rushed out the door." People are being asked to sign off on things they normally wouldn't. She added that even vaxxed employees are very uncomfortable with the process they are seeing and are willing to walk away (from their jobs) because they think something is wrong.

She also said that she and other employees were shocked to see the vials of COVID vaccine "glowing." They had never seen this before. She was told by a friend who had worked there for a very long time that the people who work in the mixing department at Pfizer normally know what the ingredients are that they are mixing. But that is not the case with the COVID vaccines. Not being told what all the ingredients are has made Pfizer employees skeptical, she said.

Based on the above information, do you believe the vaccines are safe and should continue to be given? If so, how many more deaths and serious injuries do you think are "acceptable" to the public before being pulled off the market? Consider that in light of the fact that the government has totally ignored its own standard of 50 deaths associated with a drug as being the threshold for a recall.

---

[328] Craig Paardekooper, "COVID Vax Variability Between Lots," https://www.bitchute.com/video/4HlIyBmOEJeY/ (Dec. 15, 2021)

[329] See also, Ramola D., "Super Toxic Batches and Variability in Vaccines," https://everydayconcerned.net/tag/team-enigma/ (Jan. 11, 2022)

[330] Personal communication from Sasha Latypova to Sally Saxon, Nov. 2022.

[331] https://dailyexpose.uk/2021/11/01/dr-mike-yeadon-just-when-you-though-things-couldnt-get-any-worse/ (Nov. 1, 2021)

[332] Dr. Michael Yeadon presentation, https://odysee.com/@Quasar:3/Mike-Yeadon-Testimony-for-the-Grand-Jury:9 (testimony date: Feb. 4, 2022)

[333] Interview by Brannon Howse, https://www.worldviewweekend.com/tv/video/pfizer-whistleblower-melissa-mcatee-vaccine-glowing-and-what-happened-when-she-confronted (Oct. 19, 2021).

PART 3

INEFFECTIVENESS and OTHER IMPACTS OF THE VACCINES

"When the whole world is running towards the cliff, he who is running in the opposite direction appears to have lost his mind."

C.S. Lewis

ACCESS TO HYPERLINKS *of* ONLINE REFERENCES

For easy access to hyperlinks for all of the online references cited in this book, use the QR code on the left or the "Endnotes Hyperlinks" button at www.SallySaxon.com.

Chapter 24
General Issues Concerning Effectiveness

*"Truth does not mind being questioned.
A lie does not like being challenged."*

Author Unknown

Part 3 provides an overview of several issues relating to the effectiveness of the COVID vaccines. It discusses ways in which the data and definitions have been manipulated to misrepresent and hide the vaccines' true effectiveness. It addresses the high number of breakthrough cases, a comparison of natural vs. vaccine immunity, and risk/benefit analyses. It also briefly addresses the issue of whether the vaccines are causing the variants, and reports from other sources showing serious adverse impacts, including autopsy and embalmers' findings, and unprecedented increases in life insurance and disability claims. This part concludes with a discussion of "who needs to be protected from whom," including the problem of shedding (or transmission), and the second of three reasons that answer the question of why many have not heard this information before.

It should be kept in mind, as explained in Part 1 by Dr. Toby Rogers and Dr. Michael Yeadon, the former Pfizer V.P. and scientist, that SARS-CoV-2 was never a good candidate for a vaccine in the first place. Viruses that evolve quickly mutate too fast for a vaccine to be effective because vaccine development cannot keep up with the rapid mutations. That is why, Rogers said, there has never been a vaccine for the common cold, which is part of the coronavirus family – "all previous attempts to develop a vaccine against coronaviruses have failed (they never made it out of animal trials because the animals died during challenge trials or were injured by the vaccine)."[334] Rogers also explains some of the negative consequences of trying to vaccinate against a rapidly mutating virus:

"Original antigenic sin, antibody-dependent enhancement, and the possibility of accelerating the evolution of the virus in ways that make it more virulent (and even more resistant to vaccination) are some known negative impacts."[335]

Perhaps this explains the revealing admissions by Dr. Deborah Birx, former White House COVID response coordinator, who said in an interview on July 22, 2022:[336]

> **"I knew these vaccines were not going to protect against infection. And I think we overplayed the vaccines**, and it made people then worry that it's not going to protect against severe disease and hospitalization. It will. But let's be very clear: **50% of the people who died from the Omicron surge were older, vaccinated."**

When did she first discover that the shots would not protect against infection? Did she tell that to the American public and the medical community as soon as she knew?

Though she still claims the shots protect against severe disease and hospitalization, you be the judge of that from the data in this book. At least Birx acknowledged that half of the people who died of Omicron were vaccinated. *How many of the other half might have actually been vaccinated as well with at least one shot but were counted as "unvaccinated" because they died within the 14-day window in which the CDC still deemed them to be unvaccinated?* (See discussion below) We will never know. In any event, since she acknowledged that the vaccinated had the same risk of death as the unvaccinated, her admission is an acknowledgement that the vaccine did not really make a difference regarding deaths from Omicron. As the data below will show, as time goes on, the vaccinated have fared increasingly worse, not just against COVID, but against other diseases as well. That is because of the damage the shots have done to the immune system and other systems and organs, as discussed in Part 2.

No wonder that Dr. Ryan Cole, a board-certified pathologist trained at the Mayo Clinic, has confirmed the obvious: "It doesn't matter if they're effective if they are not safe."[337] Nevertheless, it is still important to look at several issues concerning effectiveness, for at least a couple reasons: 1) to show the serious discrepancies between the official narrative and the

GENERAL ISSUES CONCERNING EFFECTIVENESS

data, including the government's own; and 2) to expose additional serious misrepresentations, withholding of critical information, and other ways the data has been manipulated.

It is also important to keep in mind that the so-called "fact-checkers" will always attack data or information that is contrary to the official narrative. The authors welcome corrections to any data or other information that is determined by credible sources to be inaccurate. However, one of the foundational issues for all readers throughout this book is: *"whose report will you believe?"*

CDC's Very Misleading Definitions of "Vaccinated" and "Unvaccinated"

To accurately assess the effectiveness of the COVID vaccines and their harmful impacts, it is important to know the CDC's definitions of who is considered to be vaccinated and who is not. You would think that should be a very easy and straightforward issue, but not according to the CDC. The CDC website says a person is not "fully vaccinated "until *2 weeks after* their second dose in a 2-dose series, such as the Pfizer or Moderna vaccines, or 2 weeks after a single-dose vaccine...."[338] However, the CDC website states that "fully vaccinated" is a term that defines only those who have had the full primary series, whether one or two shots. It does not include boosters. Dr. Joseph Mercola explains this definition:

> "In other words, if you've received one dose of Pfizer or Moderna and develop symptomatic COVID-19, get admitted to the hospital and/or die from COVID, you're counted as an unvaccinated case. If you've received two doses and get ill within 14 days, you're still counted as an unvaccinated case." [339]

"Fully vaccinated" is to be distinguished from "up to date" which refers to those who have had all available booster shots.[340] Elsewhere on the CDC website, it defines a "vaccine breakthrough infection" as:

> *"the detection of SARS-CoV-2 RNA or antigen in a respiratory specimen collected from a person ≥14 days after they have completed all recommended doses of a U.S. Food and Drug Administration (FDA)-authorized COVID-19 vaccine."*[341]

That definition would appear to include boosters. Therefore, we can also say: if you have had the primary series but have not had all available boosters, you are still considered "unvaccinated," even if more than 14 days have passed since your last shot.

Mercola noted yet another way that the CDC manipulates the data:

> "The CDC also hides vaccine failures and props up the 'pandemic of the unvaccinated' narrative by only counting breakthrough cases that result in hospitalization or death. In other words, if you got your second COVID shot more than 14 days ago and you develop symptoms, you do not count as a breakthrough case unless you're admitted to the hospital and/or die from COVID-19 in the hospital, even if you test positive." [342]

Some may argue that the above definition of "fully vaccinated" is justified because it takes several days for the shots to reach maximum effectiveness. However, Dr. Sherri Tenpenny, who has been warning about these shots since 2020 even before the rollout, has stated that this new definition of "vaccinated" was announced only after the CDC realized so many deaths were occurring within 14 days of people getting the shots.[343] In December 2021, Dr. Peter McCullough reported that *half of the deaths were occurring within 48 hours of injection, and 80% of the deaths within one week.*[344] The data presented in Part 2 by attorney Thomas Renz showed that *in the first 6 months of the rollout, 50,000 people in the age 65+ demographic died within 14 days of the 1st or 2nd shot.* [345] You may see others who report lower figures for the numbers or percentage of people who have died within the first week or two after vaccination. However, regardless of what the most accurate percentages are in the first two days or within the first or second week, the point is that there has been and apparently continues to be a substantial wave of deaths within 14 days of vaccination, especially in the first week. That is borne out by the unusual number of deaths of young Canadian doctors reported in Part 2, who died within days of their mandated 4th shot. However, do not forget the discovery of the apparent "5-month" spike, also discussed in Part 2, which showed a second wave of deaths that occurs around 5 months post-vax. Moreover, with new formulations of the shots now being administered, only time will tell what new trends may appear.

What also makes this definition with the "14 day" qualifying language **totally misleading** is that it skews the data in a way that *makes it impossible for anyone to know how many who were counted as*

GENERAL ISSUES CONCERNING EFFECTIVENESS

"unvaccinated" had actually received one or more shots. To the general public, "unvaccinated" means a person has not had any COVID shots at all. They would **not** consider as "unvaccinated" a person who had received even one shot, or someone who had the full primary series and then died within 14 days of injection. In addition, according to Dr. Deborah Viglione, hospitals often had their own definitions of "unvaccinated." One local hospital in her area recorded people as "unvaccinated" if they had not received a COVID shot within the past 7 days! This appears to be a deliberate attempt to manipulate their data to show that almost all of their COVID patients were unvaccinated. It also had its effect on their employees who said that this was a "pandemic of the unvaccinated" – that all of the people they were seeing were unvaccinated.

Another possible reason why vaccinated persons may show up as unvaccinated is that it depends on where they received their shot(s). Apparently, their vaccination record is not in their electronic medical record unless it was sent to their primary care physician.[346]

Problems Relating to the Reliability of U.S. Data

Issues like those discussed above obviously create significant problems in obtaining reliable data. Another aspect of the unreliability of the U.S. data was reported in a *ProPublica* article[347] dated August 20, 2021, that a few months earlier, on May 1:

> "as the new variant found a foothold in the U.S. — the Centers for Disease Control and Prevention mostly stopped tracking COVID-19 in vaccinated people, also known as breakthrough cases, unless the illness was severe enough to cause hospitalization or death.
>
> Individual states now set their own criteria for collecting data on breakthrough cases, resulting in a muddled grasp of COVID-19's impact, leaving experts in the dark as to the true number of infections among the vaccinated, whether or not vaccinated people can develop long-haul illness, and the risks to unvaccinated children as they return to school."

An article in *The Epoch Times* also reported on the problem of getting reliable data because of the CDC's definition of who is considered to be unvaccinated. It reports that "**the Centers for Disease Control and**

Prevention (CDC) have publicly acknowledged that they do not have accurate data." [348] That is based on a report by the Associated Press (AP) that the CDC had "not estimated what percentage of hospitalizations and deaths are in fully vaccinated people, *citing limitations in the data."* [349] **That then raises the question:** *who is responsible for creating the limitations in the data that are preventing accurate tracking and reporting? Who created the confusing and misleading definitions? With all of the current capabilities of technology, and the untold millions of dollars available to the government, why are they not able to track these categories of data?*

Without more details about how many shots, if any, people have had, it is impossible to know how effective these shots have really been. One doctor who spoke to *The Epoch Times* said that all we do know is that "the vaccines are not as effective as public health officials told us they would be. 'This is a product that's not doing what it's supposed to do. It's supposed to stop transmission of this virus and it's not doing that.'" [350]

More recently it was reported that it is ***not*** that the CDC ***stopped tracking*** the breakthrough data, but only that ***they chose not to release it***, allegedly out of concern that they would be "misinterpreted,"[351] as reported in Part 2. *Again, does the CDC think that health care professionals are not smart enough to properly interpret the data? Or are they afraid that the alleged "misinformation spreaders" may expose the discrepancies between the data and the official narrative?*

Dr. Mercola points out yet another way the CDC has been manipulating data, concerning the cycle threshold (Ct) at which the PCR tests were run, as discussed in Part 1:

> "Originally, the CDC recommended labs use a CT [cycle threshold] of 40 when testing for SARS-CoV-2 infection. This, despite using a CT above 35 was known to create a false positive rate of 97%. By using an exaggerated CT, healthy people were deemed stricken with COVID-19.
>
> "In May 2021, the CDC lowered the CT from 40 to 28 or lower — but only when doing PCR testing on individuals who have received the COVID jab. Unvaccinated were still tested using a CT of 40. The end result is obvious: 'Vaccinated' individuals became far less likely to test positive for SARS-CoV-2

GENERAL ISSUES CONCERNING EFFECTIVENESS

infection while unvaccinated were still exceedingly getting false positives..."[352]

This kind of manipulation presents yet another factor that hinders an accurate determination of the effectiveness of the vaccines. It also raises questions such as: *will this kind of manipulation ever stop?*

---

[334] Toby Rogers, Ph.D., https://brownstone.org/articles/the-fdas-future-framework-for-covid-vaccines-is-reckless-plan/ (June 22, 2022)

[335] Id.

[336] Dr. Deborah Birx interviewed by Neil Cavuto, https://www.foxnews.com/media/dr-deborah-birx-knew-covid-vaccines-not-protect-against-infection (July 22, 2022)

[337] Dr. Ryan Cole interviewed by Steve Kirsch, https://rumble.com/v1fsq9h-ryan-cole-on-how-to-identify-a-person-killed-by-the-covid-vaccine.html (Aug. 12, 2022)

[338] "When You've Been Fully Vaccinated," https://www.cdc.gov/coronavirus/2019-ncov/vaccines/fully-vaccinated_archived.html (updated Oct. 15, 2021) (last accessed May 6, 2022)

[339] Dr. Joseph Mercola, "Shockingly, CDC Now Lists Vaccinated Deaths as Unvaccinated," https://takecontrol.substack.com/p/cdc-lists-vaccinated-deaths-as-unvaccinated (Sept. 15, 2021)

[340] https://www.cdc.gov/coronavirus/2019-ncov/vaccines/faq.html

[341] COVID-19 Vaccine Breakthrough Infections Reported to CDC – United States, January 1, 2021-April 30, 2021, https://www.cdc.gov/mmwr/volumes/70/wr/mm7021e3.htm (May 28, 2021) (last accessed Nov.2, 2022)

[342] Dr. Joseph Mercola, "Shockingly, CDC Now Lists Vaccinated Deaths as Unvaccinated," https://takecontrol.substack.com/p/cdc-lists-vaccinated-deaths-as-unvaccinated (Sept. 15, 2021)

[343] Dr. Sherri Tenpenny interviewed by Reiner Fuellmich, https://thereisnopandemic.net/2022/04/22/why-the-shots-cannot-be-detoxed-from-the-body-drs-sherri-tenpenny-reiner-fuellmich/#comment-3833 (April 22, 2022)

[344] https://dareseektruth.com/dr-peter-mccullough/

[345] https://renz-law.com/special-notice-regarding-evidentiary-findings-related-to-the-official-renz-law-covid-19-investigation/

[346] Dr. Joseph Mercola, "Shockingly, CDC Now Lists Vaccinated Deaths as Unvaccinated," https://takecontrol.substack.com/p/cdc-lists-vaccinated-deaths-as-unvaccinated (Sept. 15, 2021)

[347] Jenny Deam and Bianca Fortis, https://www.propublica.org/article/the-cdc-only-tracks-a-fraction-of-breakthrough-covid-19-infections-even-as-cases-surge (Aug. 6, 2021)

[348] Jennifer Margulis, https://www.theepochtimes.com/mkt_morningbrief/whos-really-being-hospitalized_3963392.html (Aug. 30, 2021, updated Sept. 8, 2021)

[349] Carla K. Johnson and Mike Stobbe, "Nearly all COVID deaths in the US are now among unvaccinated," https://apnews.com/article/coronavirus-pandemic-health-941fcf43d9731c76c16e7354f5d5e187 (June 29, 2021)

[350] Jennifer Margulis, https://www.theepochtimes.com/mkt_morningbrief/whos-really-being-hospitalized_3963392.html (Aug. 30, 2021, updated Sept. 8, 2021)

[351] Apoorva Mandavilli, https://www.nytimes.com/2022/02/20/health/covid-cdc-data.html (Feb 20, updated Feb 22, 2022)

[352] Dr. Joseph Mercola, "Older Than 50: 60% Who Die From COVID Are Double Vaxxed," https://takecontrol.substack.com/p/fully-vaccinated-covid-deaths (Aug. 30, 2021)

Chapter 25
Breakthrough Cases

Breakthrough cases became inevitable as the effectiveness of the shots waned and new variants emerged that the original formulations of the vaccines no longer protected against. Yet on July 21, 2021, Joe Biden said in a townhall meeting: "If you're vaccinated, you're not going to be hospitalized, not going to the ICU unit, and not going to die. You're not going to get COVID if you have these vaccinations."[353]

One of numerous examples revealing early on that the vaccines were not nearly as effective as people thought is what happened in Massachusetts in the summer of 2021: "A CDC investigation of an outbreak in Barnstable County, Massachusetts, between July 6, 2021, through July 25, 2021, found 74% of those who received a diagnosis of COVID-19, and 80% of hospitalizations, were among the fully vaccinated...."[354]

Many sources agree that vaccine data from Israel is considered to be a model.[355] Based on a report published in August 2021 in Israel:

> "data show those who have received the COVID jab are 6.72 times more likely to get infected than people with natural immunity.
>
> "The fully 'vaccinated' also made up the bulk of serious cases and COVID-related deaths in July 2021...
>
> "According to Science magazine, breakthrough cases are now multiplying at breakneck speed. 'There are so many breakthrough infections that they dominate and most of the hospitalized patients are actually vaccinated...'"

Data from the UK revealed that "As of August 15, 2021: 68% of COVID patients admitted to hospital in the U.K. who were over the age of 50 had received one or two doses ... "[356] On August 21, Dr. Peter McCullough reported data from Israel which showed that through July 2021, over 80% of the population was vaccinated, yet of the 15,634 COVID cases recorded, 86% were among the fully vaxxed.[357]

An article published in November 2021 entitled "Statistical Proof that COVID-19 Vaccines are Worse than Ineffective—They Are Causing Most of the COVID-19 Hospitalizations" presents many examples of breakthrough cases, even places where vaccinated persons represented up to 100% of hospitalizations for COVID.[358] It also reveals that UK government data was showing that the 5% loss of efficacy *per week* they were seeing actually continues past zero. That means **"the vaccine *increases* the likelihood of COVID-19."** That is called "negative efficacy."

Even the data concerning the effectiveness of the COVID shots in children have been shown to demonstrate very poor results, as well as how nonsensical government policies are around this issue. *The New York Times* reported on February 28, 2022, while still claiming the vaccine prevented severe illness in children, it "offers virtually no protection against infection, even within a month after full immunization…" That conclusion was based on data from a study by the New York State Department of Health which showed that after 2 months, efficacy for 5 to 11-year-olds had sunk to 12%. Yet the Department still concluded that this age group should get the shots because they are supposedly "protective against severe disease."[359] **Does that make any sense?** According to that *NYT* article, a lower dose was given to the younger children which could account for the very low effectiveness. ***But the better question is not: should the younger children then be given a higher dose or more boosters? Rather, it is: do children even need a vaccine in the first place?*** As reported in Part 1, the CDC's own data infection fatality data showed the survival rate from COVID for children under 18 was 99.997% based on the protection offered by their own natural immune system.[360]

Prof. Jacob Giris, director of Israel's Ichilov Hospital's coronavirus ward, said in February 2022 that most of their cases had had at least three COVID shots, and the vaccinated accounted for 70-80% of their cases. *"So, the vaccine has no significance regarding severe illness,"* he said.[361]

A report with more recent data from the 1st quarter of 2022 presents results that totally undermine the "pandemic of the unvaccinated" narrative. Official data of the UK Health Security Agency:

"confirms the fully vaccinated population accounted for a shocking 92% of all Covid-19 deaths across England throughout March [2022], but what's even more shocking is that 82% of those deaths were among the triple vaccinated population.

"But something even stranger than this is also occurring. Covid-19 is currently on the rise again across the UK, but the data confirms cases, hospitalisations and deaths are only rising among the triple vaccinated population, whereas they are declining significantly among the unvaccinated population." [362]

That same report shows that the total number of hospitalizations among the vaccinated during February and March 2022 far surpassed those among the unvaccinated, as shown in Table 14 below. By far, the triple-vaxxed represented the vast majority of the total.

Table 14.[363] UK Health Security Agency data for England (Feb./March 2022)

HOSPITALIZATIONS Time period	Unvaxxed	Triple vaxxed only	Total Vaxxed 1,2, or 3 doses	% of totals represented by total # of vaxxed
1/24 to 2/20/22	2,341	4,936	6,889	75%
2/28 to 3/27/22	2,065	6,750	8,261	80%
TOTAL for both periods	**4,406**	**11,686**	**15,150**	
DEATHS Time period				
1/24 to 2/20/22	559	3,120	4,302	88.5%
2/28 to 3/27/22	321	3,054	3,736	92.3%
TOTAL for both periods	**880**	**6,174**	**8,038**	

The total number of COVID *cases* for those same time periods reflects the same pattern. **All of the data together for the number of cases, hospitalizations and deaths reveal that the more doses a person gets, the more likely they are to get COVID, be hospitalized or die.** However, *do we really know the "breakthrough" hospitalizations and deaths were actually due to COVID-19 and not to the shots?*

The same trend is revealed by the official data for Canada as well. Tables 15 and 16 below show the data for COVID cases, hospitalizations and deaths in early 2022. Note the percentages represented by the triple vaxxed alone, and the total percentage in each category that all vaxxed represent. As with the England data above, the same question arises as to whether all the deaths attributed to COVID were actually due to COVID or may have been from the shots themselves.

Table 15: [364] COVID-19 Case, Hospitalization & Death Data: Canada (Feb. 21– May 29, 2022) (Based on data from the Government of Canada Daily Epidemiology Update)

Feb. 21 – May 29 2022	Unvaxxed	1 dose	2 doses	3 doses	Total vaxxed – all doses (& % of all, incl. unvaxxed)
Cases	52,884	11,211	138,086	227,154	376,451 (88% of all)
Hospitalizations	5,615	855	6,489	12,373	19,717 (78% of all)
Deaths	1,158	135	1,174	2,487	3,796 (77% of all)

Table 16 below shows the same data points for only the last part of the above time period, plus an extra week, showing that the numbers grew progressively worse over time. Note the increased percentages that vaccinated persons represent in all categories.

Table 16: [365] COVID-19 Case, Hospitalization & Death Data: Canada (May 1– June 5, 2022). (Based on data from the Government of Canada Daily Epidemiology Update)

May 1 – June 5, 2022	Unvaxxed	1 dose	2 doses	3 doses	Total vaxxed – all doses (& % of all, including unvaxxed)
Cases	8,436	4,381	40,327	74,118	118,826 (93%)
Hospitalizations	1,065	242	1,728	4,590	6,560 (86%)
Deaths	235	41	318	1,113	1,472 (86%)

BREAKTHROUGH CASES

Breakthrough cases started emerging at least as early as mid-2021. What have we learned since then? Hopefully, at the very least, the above data show us that the "pandemic of the unvaccinated" was all propaganda to shame and demonize the unvaccinated and encourage people that the "patriotic" and "right" thing to do was to get the shots.

---

[353] Alexandra Jaffe and Aamer Madhani, https://www.cbs8.com/article/news/health/coronavirus/vaccine/biden-covid-vaccine-drive/507-6f482433-d3cf-41ee-a09d-b7f01e1436bd (July 21, 2021)

[354] Dr. Joseph Mercola, "Shockingly, CDC Now Lists Vaccinated Deaths as Unvaccinated," https://takecontrol.substack.com/p/cdc-lists-vaccinated-deaths-as-unvaccinated (Sept. 15, 2021) Other sources, including CDC documents, are cited in that article.

[355] See several sources cited in Dr. Joseph Mercola, "60% of Those 50 or Older Who Die from COVID are Double Vaxxed," https://takecontrol.substack.com/p/fully-vaccinated-covid-deaths (Aug. 30, 2021).

[356] Id.

[357] Dr. Peter McCullough interviewed by Stew Peters, https://www.redvoicemedia.com/video/2021/08/vaccine-failure-dr-peter-mccullough-reveals-data-damning-to-efficacy-narrative/ (August 17, 2021)

[358] Edward Hendrie https://greatmountainpublishing.com/2021/11/12/statistical-proof-that-covid-19-vaccines-are-worse-than-ineffective-they-are-causing-most-of-the-covid-19-hospitalizations/ (Nov.12, 2021)

[359] Dr. Meryl Nass, https://thepulse.one/2022/05/02/the-covid-vaccine-narrative-has-sunk-and-the-powers-that-be-have-stopped-trying-to-hide-it/ (May 2, 2022)

[360] https://web.archive.org/web/20201127224157/https://www.cdc.gov/coronavirus/2019-ncov/hcp/planning-scenarios.html

[361] https://www.israelnationalnews.com/news/321674 (Feb. 3, 2022)

[362] https://dailyexpose.uk/2022/04/12/distracted-boris-kyiv-fully-vaccinated-92-percent-covid-deaths/ (April 12, 2022)

[363] Id.

[364] https://expose-news.com/2022/06/15/vaccinated-4-in-5-covid-deaths-canada-since-feb/?cmid=cd02f5ae-8cfc-48d8-97d2-a6cc37f11d25 (June 15, 2022)

[365] https://expose-news.com/2022/06/22/trudeau-panics-9-in-10-covid-deaths-fully-vaccinated/ (June 22, 2022)

Chapter 26
Boosters and Variants

The Waning of Vaccine Protection Gave Rise to the Boosters

Dr. Peter McCullough, who has served on many review boards, including for vaccines, stated in December 2021: *"Vaccines aren't viable if they can't last a year! The minimum criteria...is 50% coverage and it must last one year. These [COVID shots] aren't cutting it. None of them are viable to be commercial products."*[366] The FDA issued a statement based on its June 2020 Guidance document that it "would expect that a COVID-19 vaccine would prevent disease or decrease its severity in at least 50% of people who are vaccinated."[367]

There are many reports that show a high rate of efficacy for the first half of 2021, but that early data became rather irrelevant as the months passed, as Delta appeared in mid-2021 and the scenario started changing. One Swedish study that was published in October 2021 covered the period from January 12, 2021 to October 4, 2021.[368] It involved 842,974 pairs of people in which one person got two shots and the other received none. The study found the Pfizer shot declined in effectiveness against infection from 92% from day 15 through 30 to only 47% during the period from days 121 through 180, and from day 211 on, "no effectiveness could be detected." Effectiveness "waned slightly slower" for the Moderna shot, estimated at 59% "from day 181 and onwards" (though the study only studied the period up to October 4, so its effectiveness beyond that date is not known). The authors of the study interpreted their results as follows:

> "effectiveness against symptomatic Covid-19 infection wanes progressively over time across all subgroups, but at different rate [*sic*] according to type of vaccine, and faster for men and older frail individuals. The effectiveness against severe illness remains high through 9 months, although not for men, older frail individuals, and individuals with comorbidities. This

strengthens the evidence-based rationale for administration of a third booster dose."

However, their suggested rationale is not the only possibility. *Might an alternative interpretation be this: "Since the first two shots were not very effective, why should anyone think that a third one would somehow last a lot longer?"*

Interestingly, the above study showed that the Pfizer's vaccine effectiveness had declined to less than 47% by day 121 (less than the FDA's threshold of 50%). The start date of the study was January 12, 2021, so 4 months later would have been April 2021. Pfizer CEO Bourla had already announced on April 1, 2021 that a booster would likely be needed 6-12 months after the primary series of shots, and then annually thereafter.[369] That was shortly before the FDA announced that it had "approved" Pfizer's Comirnaty product on August 23, 2021. (There has been some controversy over whether the action taken by FDA that day constituted a full approval and licensure, but that issue is outside the scope of this book.) *What efficacy data did Pfizer present to the FDA in its application for licensure?* The FDA's minimum efficacy rate is 50%, but according to the Swedish study, Pfizer's effectiveness had waned to 47% in only 4 months, by April. The Swedish study did not come out until after the FDA's decision in August, so it would be interesting to compare the data from the large Swedish study with the data Pfizer gave to the FDA when it submitted its application for licensure of the Comirnaty vaccine.

On June 29, 2021, Anthony Fauci said in an interview that the new variant (Delta) was a "game-changer" for the unvaccinated. He said that those who were vaccinated were "doing fine," and that "if you're vaccinated, you're in …quite good shape. If you're not vaccinated, you're at significant risk."[370] *Then why are the data showing that the vast majority of COVID cases, hospitalizations and deaths are among the vaccinated?* The very next day Dr. Peter McCullough said in an interview:[371] "It is very clear from the UK Technical Briefing[372] that was published June 18 [2021] that **the vaccine provides no protection against the Delta variant**." The reason, McCullough explained, is that "The Delta variant contains three different mutations, all in the spike protein. This allows this variant to evade the immune responses in those who have received the COVID jabs, but not those who have natural immunity, which is much broader." ***Whose report should you believe?***

A study published in August 2021[373] showed that in June-July, after Delta became the predominant variant, effectiveness of the Pfizer and Moderna shots had waned to 53.1% among certain U.S. nursing home and long-term care facility residents, one of the most vulnerable populations. The CEO of Moderna was already acknowledging by early that same month that a third shot would probably be necessary to deal with the Delta variant.[374] However, the first two shots were ineffective against the Delta variant since they were directed at the original Wuhan spike protein. The Delta variant had mutated too much for the vaccine to have any effectiveness at all. ***Why would a third shot of an expired vaccine be effective if the first two were not?***

A paper entitled "Increases in cases of COVID-19 are unrelated to levels of vaccination across 68 countries and 2,947 counties in the United States" was published in September 2021.[375] The authors found "no significant signaling of COVID-19 cases decreasing with higher percentages of population fully vaccinated." It also noted that "the trend line suggests a marginally positive association such that countries with higher percentage of population fully vaccinated have higher COVID-19 cases per one million people."

On September 22, 2021 the FDA extended Pfizer's EUA to include a booster shot at least 6 months after the primary series for certain groups of people, those 65+ and 18 to 64-year-olds in certain risk categories.[376] McCullough reported that as of the end of October 2021, there were "22 studies showing the shots' efficacy against all variants rapidly wane over the course of three to six months, eventually hitting zero."[377] One of those was the Swedish study mentioned above. By early January 2022, the CEO of Pfizer acknowledged that their two primary doses were not enough against Omicron and a booster would be needed.[378] Fortunately for Pfizer, but unfortunately for the public, the FDA had already extended Pfizer's EUA to include the booster. In contrast, McCullough said that those who had already had COVID have natural immunity that does not diminish like the protection claimed to be provided by the vaccines.[379]

Then on March 29, 2022, the FDA authorized a second Pfizer booster (a fourth shot) after at least 4 months following the first booster, but only for those over 50 and those with certain kinds of immunocompromise.[380]

Does this mean that they are going to recommend boosters every 4 months now, at least for certain large groups? Did not the Pfizer CEO say in April of 2021 that after the first booster, additional boosters would likely only be needed annually? Is there any end in sight for COVID booster shots? Endless boosters certainly bode well for the bottom line of the vaccine manufacturers' financial statements, especially since the shots are being paid for by the government.

Americans should be glad – at least for the time being – that they do not live in Germany, where it was announced by the Federal Health Minister in August 2022 that Germans would have to receive COVID boosters every 3 months to be considered "vaccinated," despite a decline in COVID numbers![381] The vaccinated would be exempt from some of the new "freedom-crushing laws."

Canadians may be facing a similar situation. An article dated September 2, 2022, announced that a similar proposal had been made by Canada's National Advisory Committee on Immunization, that "shots may be warranted" every 90 days, due to waning efficacy.[382] The Canadian Department of Health had announced just weeks earlier that boosters at 9-month intervals would be enough, but the deputy chief public health officer said that due to waning immunity, a booster even every six months was not sufficient. The Health Minister explained that being "fully vaccinated" was not good enough – people had to be "up-to-date" in their vaccinations.

Dr. Toby Rogers noted that when the FDA's expert advisory committee (VRBPAC) met for the first time to discuss the "Future Framework" on April 6, 2022 "*all of* the committee members agreed that COVID-19 shots are not working, that boosting multiple times a year was not feasible, and that the shots need to be reformulated."[383] As Rogers explained:

> "Over half a billion doses have been injected into Americans in the past 17 months and these shots have made no discernible impact on the course of the pandemic. Far more Americans have died of coronavirus since the introduction of the shots than before they were introduced."

That led to the FDA's action in late June to start implementing the new "Future Framework" scheme, explained in greater detail in Part 2. Under that framework, the vaccine manufacturers could get authorization for any newly reformulated COVID vaccines **without any new clinical trials**.

That enabled Pfizer and Moderna to continue making tens of billions of dollars in annual revenue without having to face new clinical trials or take the risk that they would not pass regulatory review. Since the clinical trials for the original vaccines were deficient in many ways and the regulatory review was quite lax, as reported by Sasha Latypova, Brook Jackson and others in Part 2, it is doubtful that new trials would have been subject to a truly objective and rigorous review anyway. But doing away with the clinical trial requirement only seems to have formalized the deficient and lax process already being followed by the vaccine manufacturers and their "captured" regulatory agencies that are supposed to oversee them.

Nevertheless, despite the FDA advisory committee's acknowledgements that the shots were not working and boosting multiple times a year was not feasible, in July 2022 Anthony Fauci said he thought Americans 5 to 50 years old should be authorized for a second booster. His reason was that it may have been a long time since many people got their first one (after their primary series), and it is likely that their immunity was waning.[384] After Fauci announced his support for a second booster, Dr. Robert Malone warned of the prospect of immune imprinting. He said: "I couldn't design a vaccine if I wanted to, to be more likely to drive immune imprinting." [385] That "refers to a phenomenon whereby initial exposure to a virus strain may prevent the body from producing enough neutralizing antibodies against a new viral strain."

Can you identify any other vaccine that required a booster within one year, and then another booster within just several months? Neither the American public nor the medical community was warned at the beginning that multiple and seemingly endless boosters might be required. *Does not the need for continual boosters demonstrate how ineffective these shots have been?*

What makes the booster strategy even worse is that most people do not know that "SARS-CoV-2 mutates at a rate that is two to 10 times faster than the influenza virus, and these mutations can considerably reduce vaccine effectiveness."[386] It appears that the real problem here is the government's continued refusal to acknowledge that a vaccine is not the appropriate response to a situation like this in the first place when there is such rapid mutation. Especially if it mutates 2 to 10 times faster than the flu, *how is it possible to stay ahead of the curve?* **With each passing day, it appears that the government's response (driven by Big Pharma) makes less and less sense. It appears to fit the proverbial** definition of "insanity"– doing the same thing over and over and expecting a different result.

On January 11, 2022, the World Health Organization's Technical Advisory Group on COVID-19 Vaccine Composition issued a warning: "a vaccination strategy based on repeated booster doses of the original vaccine composition is unlikely to be appropriate or sustainable." [387] Around that same time, it was reported that the European Union (EU) regulators warned:

> "frequent COVID boosters could risk overloading the immune system and said there is currently no data to support repeated doses. This comes a month after the regulators said it made sense to 'administer COVID-19 vaccine boosters as early as three months after the initial two-shot regimen,' among concerns over the Omicron variant." [388]

Do you think it is time to take a few steps back and re-consider what is really going on with the prolongation of the COVID "pandemic" and the need for any more COVID shots for anyone of any age? *Remember way back when we were told that vaccines were the only way out of the pandemic? Yet more than two and a half years later, are we really any closer to the end when those pushing the boosters do not appear to have any end in sight? Have the vaccines really contributed anything at all to public health, as the excess mortality rate (NOT a result of COVID itself) is increasing, especially among younger, relatively healthy people?*

When Anthony Fauci and the Pfizer CEO both come down with COVID even after 4 shots each, what are we to make of that?

Are the Vaccines Actually Causing the Variants?

Many experts have warned that the vaccines are likely causing the variants. Among them is the late Dr. Luc Montagnier, a French Nobel Prize winner in Medicine for discovering HIV. An article about an interview he did shortly before his death reports the following:[389]

> "he states that the mass vaccination program is an 'enormous mistake' and a 'medical error' because 'it is clear that the new variants are created by antibody-mediated selection due to the vaccination.'"

He was saying that the vaccines were creating the variants. *How much weight does the opinion of a distinguished Nobel Prize recipient carry?*

Dr. Jessica Rose is the Canadian researcher cited in Parts 1 and 2 who has a Bachelor's Degree in Applied Mathematics, a Master's in Immunology, a Ph.D. in Computational Biology and two Post-Doctoral degrees in Molecular Biology and Biochemistry. She has studied Israel's data, since Israel was one of the first countries to have the highest rate of vaccination. Based on the clusters of data around the time the vaccines started, she observed:

> "Israel is one of the most injected countries and it appears from the data that this represents a clear failure of these products to provide protective immunity against emergent variants and to prevent transmission, regardless of how many additional shots administered. And this begs the question as to whether these injection rollouts are driving the emergence of the new variants. There is clear and present danger of the emergence of these variants of concern if we continue with these alleged booster shots." [390]

Dr. Toby Rogers, Ph.D., who was quoted earlier, has also indicated that one of the known negative impacts of vaccinating against a rapidly mutating virus is the "possibility of accelerating the evolution of the virus in ways that make it more virulent (and even more resistant to vaccination)…" [391]

Dr. Geert Vanden Bossche, DVM, Ph.D., a virologist and vaccine developer, has also warned that a mass vaccination campaign in the middle of a pandemic would "inevitably lead to the expansion of more infectious variants."[392] On his website is a letter he wrote to the World Health Organization on December 24, 2021, which goes beyond that statement. Part of that letter reveals the problem of going against the official narrative of the medical industrial complex. An equally important part shows that there is actually more support in the scientific community than they are willing to admit that the vaccines are causing the variants:

> "one of the most renowned vaccinologists on this planet wrote me an email saying; 'vaccinating with these vaccines would only breed new variants. But that it wouldn't make sense for me to go against the mainstream because nobody would listen to me anyway, and hopefully that second-generation vaccines would solve the problem.'"[393]

An article published by the Informed Consent Action Network (ICAN) in April 2022 further confirms the causal relationship between the vaccines and the variants: "As a number of brave immunologists and vaccinologists have been warning, the Covid-19 vaccines are going to drive new vaccine-resistant variants."[394]

ICAN has taken this issue another step, since the CDC makes the following claim on its website: **"FACT: COVID-19 vaccines do not create or cause variants of the virus that causes COVID-19. Instead, COVID-19 vaccines can help prevent new variants from emerging."**[395] Based on that claim of "fact," ICAN made two FOIA requests, each with slightly different language, asking for all documents the CDC has that support that claim. Each time the CDC's response was that they "found no records responsive" to the requests.[396] In other words, the CDC has *nothing* to support that claim which they label as "FACT!" *Did they just pull that "fact" out of thin air because they needed such a statement to support their narrative and justify more shots?* As ICAN's attorney has stated, if the CDC is making declaratory statements like that, representing certain things as "facts," they had better have evidence to back them up.[397]

How many other claims has the government made concerning "all things COVID" for which they have absolutely no supporting evidence? Does not their total lack of evidence on this point totally undermine the rationale for any boosters (aside from the data showing that those who have received the boosters are actually worse off than those who have not)?

Do you think it is time to re-think the issue of what is really causing so many variants and the justification for COVID-19 booster shots?

---

[366] Dr. Joseph Mercola summary of presentation by Dr. Peter McCullough, "What You Need to Know About the COVID Shot, and More," at COVID Symposium: A Legal Perspective (Dec. 3, 2021); https://takecontrol.substack.com/p/peter-mccullough-covid-spike-protein-lecture (Jan. 17, 2022)

[367] https://www.fda.gov/news-events/press-announcements/coronavirus-covid-19-update-fda-takes-action-help-facilitate-timely-development-safe-effective-covid (June 2020); https://www.fda.gov/media/139638/download

[368] Nordström, Peter and Ballin, Marcel and Nordström, Anna, Effectiveness of Covid-19 Vaccination Against Risk of Symptomatic Infection, Hospitalization, and Death Up to 9 Months: A Swedish Total-Population Cohort Study. Available at SSRN: https://ssrn.com/abstract=3949410 ; http://dx.doi.org/10.2139/ssrn.3949410

[369] Berkeley Lovelace, Jr., https://www.cnbc.com/2021/04/15/pfizer-ceo-says-third-covid-vaccine-dose-likely-needed-within-12-months.html (April 15, 2021)

[370] https://www.pbs.org/newshour/show/dr-fauci-on-delta-variant-booster-shots-and-masks-for-the-vaccinated (June 29, 2021)

[371] Dr. Peter McCullough interviewed by Laura Ingraham, https://covidcalltohumanity.org/2021/07/05/dont-fear-the-delta-variant-treat-it/ (June 30, 2021)

[372] https://assets.publishing.service.gov.uk/government/uploads/system/uploads/attachment_data/file/1001359/Variants_of_Concern_VOC_Technical_Briefing_16.pdf (June 18, 2021)

[373] https://www.cdc.gov/mmwr/volumes/70/wr/mm7034e3.htm

[374] https://nationalfile.com/moderna-admits-their-covid-19-vaccine-only-lasts-for-6-months-booster-jab-will-likely-be-necessary/ (Aug. 5, 2021);

[375] Subramanian, S.V., Kumar, A. Increases in COVID-19 are unrelated to levels of vaccination across 68 countries and 2947 counties in the United States. *Eur J Epidemiol* **36**, 1237–1240 (2021). https://doi.org/10.1007/s10654-021-00808-7

[376] https://www.fda.gov/news-events/press-announcements/fda-authorizes-booster-dose-pfizer-biontech-covid-19-vaccine-certain-populations (Sept. 22, 2021)

[377] Dr. Joseph Mercola summary of presentation by Dr. Peter McCullough, "What You Need to Know About the COVID Shot, and More," at COVID Symposium (above)

[378] Spencer Kimball, https://www.cnbc.com/2022/01/10/pfizer-ceo-says-two-covid-vaccine-doses-arent-enough-for-omicron.html (Jan. 10, 2022)

[379] Dr. Joseph Mercola summary of presentation by Dr. Peter McCullough, "What You Need to Know About the COVID Shot, and More," at COVID Symposium (above)

[380] https://www.fda.gov/news-events/press-announcements/coronavirus-covid-19-update-fda-authorizes-second-booster-dose-two-covid-19-vaccines-older-and

[381] Amy Mek, https://rairfoundation.com/germans-must-receive-covid-booster-every-3-months-to-qualify-as-vaccinated-video/ (Aug. 13, 2022)

[382] Matthew Horwood, https://www.westernstandard.news/business/vaccines-may-be-needed-every-90-days-federal-advisory-committee-claims/article_7df7355a-2ab4-11ed-83e1-039fe19f62a7.html (Sept. 2, 2022)

[383] Toby Rogers, PhD, https://brownstone.org/articles/the-fdas-future-framework-for-covid-vaccines-is-reckless-plan/ (June 22, 2022)

[384] Zachary Stieber, https://www.theepochtimes.com/dr-malone-warns-of-immune-imprinting-after-fauci-floats-second-booster-shots_4592464.html (July 12, 2022)

[385] Id.

[386] https://tobyrogers.substack.com/p/the-fdas-proposed-future-framework (May 31, 2022), citing Trevor Bedford's presentation April 6, 2022, at an FDA VRBPAC meeting to discuss the FutureFramework.

[387] https://www.who.int/news/item/11-01-2022-interim-statement-on-covid-19-vaccines-in-the-context-of-the-circulation-of-the-omicron-sars-cov-2-variant-from-the-who-technical-advisory-group-on-covid-19-vaccine-composition

[388] Megan Redshaw, https://childrenshealthdefense.org/defender/vaers-cdc-myocarditis-tops-list-covid-vaccine-injuries-teens/ (Jan. 14, 2022)

[389] https://rumble.com/vldilx-nobel-prize-winner-professor-luc-montagnier-says-vaccine-is-creating-varian.html (Aug, 8, 2021)

[390] Vaccines and Related Biological Products Advisory Committee – 9/17/2021, https://www.youtube.com/watch?v=WFph7-6t34M&t=15705s (Sept. 2021)

[391] Toby Rogers, PhD, https://brownstone.org/articles/the-fdas-future-framework-for-covid-vaccines-is-reckless-plan/ (June 22, 2022)

[392] https://www.voiceforscienceandsolidarity.org/videos-and-interviews/second-call-to-who-please-dont-vaccinate-against-omicron

[393] Id.

[394] https://www.icandecide.org/ican_press/the-cdcs-response-to-scientific-inquiry-because-we-said-so/ (April 29, 2022)

[395] https://www.cdc.gov/coronavirus/2019-ncov/vaccines/facts.html

[396] Zachary Stieber, https://www.theepochtimes.com/cdc-no-documents-supporting-claim-vaccines-dont-cause-variants_4464871.html (May 13, 2022)

[397] Id.

Chapter 27
Risk/Benefit Analyses

The risk/benefit analysis relates to both safety and effectiveness. Supporters of the official narrative claim that even if they get COVID, the vaccine will spare them more serious consequences. *How do they know? Where is the data, the study and the control group they are basing that claim on?* Dr. Ryan Cole has spoken directly to this issue as recently as late August 2022. He stated emphatically that "there is not one placebo-controlled, randomized controlled trial showing that that statement is true in any way, shape or form."[398] *If someone made a FOIA request for documents that support that claim, similar to ICAN's FOIA request on the issue of variants, do you think the CDC or FDA could produce any documents supporting that claim?*

The lead author of this book heard about a woman who went blind in one eye after receiving the COVID injections. There was no indication that she had any other condition that might have caused the blindness. However, she was so glad she had gotten the shots because she believed she would have gone blind in *both* eyes had she *not* gotten them! Her belief was obviously based on the claim that the shots lessen the severity of COVID disease, and that the shots could not possibly have been the cause of her blindness in the one eye. It is very sad to hear reports like that woman's, but it appears that a significant percentage of people have fallen under a similar "spell" of the official narrative which somehow prevents them from connecting the vaccines with unexpected injuries and "sudden adult deaths." It is very unfortunate that she either never knew about or did not believe in the safe and effective treatments that were available. Those treatments, used successfully by the alleged "misinformation spreading" doctors, do not carry such terrible risks.

Therefore, the question is: do these injections actually provide more benefit than risk? The data say "absolutely not." Keep in mind the criteria cited in Part 2 for determining when a drug is removed from market (upon 50 associated deaths), and how quickly the swine flu vaccine campaign was stopped after exponentially fewer adverse reactions were reported than have been reported following COVID vaccinations. *What good is any drug even if it may lessen the severity of a particular disease but causes a worse effect that leads to serious injury or death?*

Steve Kirsch, founder of the Vaccine Safety Research Foundation, whose COVID research has been cited earlier in this book, has also said that **it's "impossible" to "do any sort of risk-benefit assessment without knowing the VAERS URF [under-reporting factor]."** [399] That makes total sense. How can you make such an assessment without having the best estimates possible of the number of deaths and serious injuries from any drug? While the raw VAERS data is still good for comparison purposes, to show trends and warning signals, *it is not adequate for a risk/benefit analysis.* You have to apply a URF, as Kirsch asserts.

As indicated in Part 2, as of August 12, 2022, there had been 14,061 VAERS reports of deaths following COVID vaccinations in the U.S. alone. *Based on a URF of only 41, that would mean that more than 576,000 Americans have died following the COVID shots as of that date. If we apply the much higher URF suggested by VAERS expert Albert Benavides as discussed in Part 2, around 100, that means that a staggering number of over 1.4 million Americans have probably died following the COVID shots in just 20 months!* And that is just in the United States. Yet we are still being told, as of the fall of 2022, that the shots are safe and effective.

Remember the various problems with the numbers published in VAERS that require an increasingly high URF. For example, one is the excessive lag time in VAERS reports being published. Another is the fact that VAERS now only publishes the *initial* reports and no updated reports that might reflect that death had occurred since the time of the initial report. *Why is VAERS (i.e., the CDC) not publishing updated reports to reflect deaths or injuries that may have become permanent since the initial reports?* Would that not be a very important piece of information for everyone to know? Therefore, it is highly possible, if not likely, that a more reasonable and accurate URF is much higher than Kirsch's earlier calculation of 41, as Albert Benavides has stated. A more accurate estimate of deaths may come from the life insurance industry, which is reported below.

Other Experts' Risk/Benefit Conclusions

Many others would say, as Dr. Robert Malone has said with regard to children in Part 2 of this book, the risk/benefit analysis "is not even close." This is especially true in light of the availability of safe and effective treatments that do not carry the serious risks that these experimental injections do. Dr. Sherri Tenpenny has also concluded that there is *zero benefit, only risk* to these shots.[400] Dr. Jessica Rose, the viral immunologist and computational biologist quoted in various parts of this book made a presentation at a meeting of an FDA committee in September 2021. Her conclusion was that *the very high rate of adverse reactions to the COVID vaccines outweighed any potential public health benefit, especially for children.*[401]

A portion of one of the studies cited in Part 2, by Ronald Kostoff, et al, was based on "a non-traditional best case scenario pseudo-cost-benefit analysis of the COVID-19 inoculations for the 65+ demographic in the USA." ***That study concluded that the risks of these shots outweigh the benefits for that demographic:*** [402]

> "... our extremely conservative estimate for risk-benefit ratio is about 5/1. In plain English, people in the 65+ demographic are five times as likely to die from the inoculation as from COVID-19 under the most favorable assumptions!"

A risk/benefit study up to February 6, 2022 by Stephanie Seneff, Ph.D., and Kathy Dopp concluded: [403]

> "based on publicly available official UK and US data, all age groups under 50 years old are at greater risk of fatality after receiving a COVID-19 inoculation than an unvaccinated person is at risk of a COVID-19 death. All age groups under 80 years old have virtually no benefit from receiving a COVID-19 inoculation, and the younger ages incur significant risk. This analysis is conservative because it ignores the fact that ... vaccine-induced injuries can lead to shortened life span ..."

Dr. Toby Rogers, Ph.D., has also addressed the risk-benefit issue. Rogers says that for the COVID vaccines, "the NNTV [Number Needed to Vaccinate to save one child from a COVID-19 death] is so ridiculously high that this vaccine could not pass any honest risk-benefit analysis." His conclusion for the 5 to 11-year-old age group is: *for each child saved from death due to COVID-19, another 117 children would die following the shots.* [404] The reason the NNTV is so high for children is because the risk of them dying from COVID is almost nil in the first place, as shown in the data in Part 1. Therefore, it takes an extremely large number of children to be vaccinated to save even one child.

A very revealing analysis of data from the UK for the period Jan. 2021 – Jan. 2022 was published May 5, 2022 by Steve Kirsch.[405] Kirsch said that the "data quality here is strongly biased in favor of making the vaccine look effective." However, his conclusion is reflected in the title of his report: "New UK government data shows the vaccines kill more people than they save." He states:

> "New UK government data allows us to analyze the data in a way we couldn't before. This new analysis shows clearly that the *COVID vaccines kill more people than they save for all age groups.*
>
> "The data showed that for most age ranges, the vaccine reduced your chance of dying from COVID, but it increased your chances of dying from other causes. The former effect was smaller than the latter effect so the vaccines are nonsensical.
>
> "...Below 80, the younger you are, the more nonsensical vaccination is."

In other words, the cure is far worse than the disease. Even if different experts disagree on their estimates of the risk/benefit ratios, the point is that regardless of whose numbers are more accurate, they are all so high that none even comes close to providing a favorable risk-benefit to support these shots for any age group.

The State of Florida Department of Health studied mortality risk following mRNA COVID-19 shots. Their "Guidance for COVID-19 mRNA Vaccines" dated October 7, 2022 was based on the finding that "there is an 84% increase in the relative incidence of cardiac-related death among males 18-39 years old within 28 days following mRNA vaccination." Based on that data, the report concluded: "With a high level of global immunity to COVID-19, **the benefit of vaccination is likely outweighed by this abnormally high risk of cardiac-related death among men in this age group.**" For that reason, "The State Surgeon General now recommends against the COVID-19 mRNA vaccines for males ages 18-39 years old." [406]

In that same analysis, men over 60 were found to have a "10% increased risk of cardiac-related death within 28 days of mRNA vaccination." The analysis did not find the same increased risk from non-mRNA COVID vaccines. However, that finding does not mean that the non-mRNA shots do not also carry significant risks that the medical industrial complex has sought to hide, both from the health care community as well as from the general public.

---

[398] Dr. Ryan Cole interviewed by Red Voice Media, https://www.redvoicemedia.com/video/2022/08/dr-ryan-cole-the-jab-suppresses-the-immune-system-of-the-vaccinated/ (Aug. 26, 2022)

[399] Steve Kirsch, https://www.trialsitenews.com/a/why-wont-the-cdc-or-fda-reveal-the-vaers-urf (Oct. 25, 2021)

[400] Dr. Sherri Tenpenny Interview with Reiner Fuellmich, https://thereisnopandemic.net/2022/04/22/why-the-shots-cannot-be-detoxed-from-the-body-drs-sherri-tenpenny-reiner-fuellmich/#comment-3833 (April 22, 2022)

[401] Vaccines and Related Biological Products Advisory Committee – 9/17/2021, https://www.youtube.com/watch?v=WFph7-6t34M&t=15705s (Sept. 2021)

[402] Ronald N. Kostoff, Ph.D., et al, "Why are We Vaccinating Children Against COVID-19?" https://www.sciencedirect.com/science/article/pii/S221475002100161X#bib002 (2021)

[403] Stephanie Seneff and Kathy Dopp, "COVID-19 and All-Cause Mortality Data by Age Group Reveals Risk of Vaccine-Induced Fatality is Equal to or Greater Than the Risk of COVID Death for All Age Groups Under 80 Years Old," https://www.skirsch.com/covid/Seneff_costBenefit.pdf (Feb. 13, 2022)

[404] Dr. Toby Rogers, https://tobyrogers.substack.com/p/what-is-the-number-needed-to-vaccinate (Oct. 31, 2021)

[405] Steve Kirsch, https://stevekirsch.substack.com/p/uk-government-data-shows-nobody-should?s=w (May 5, 2022)

[406] https://floridahealthcovid19.gov/wp-content/uploads/2022/10/20221007-guidance-mrna-covid19-vaccines-doc.pdf

Chapter 28
Clinical Trial Data Reveal a Decline in Health, Not a Health Benefit

Even with more than 20 months of actual data following the COVID vaccine rollout, the clinical trial data is still significant in that it sheds light on whether this criterion required for an EUA was met or not. It also reveals certain misrepresentations or misleading use of data by the manufacturers during the trials. Part 1 in this book included an analysis of Pfizer's claim from its clinical trials that its vaccine was "95% effective." It explained that the 95% figure was extremely misleading because it only represented the relative risk reduction (RRR), not the absolute risk reduction (ARR) which was less than 1% – and which FDA guidelines say should always be included and provided to the public to aid them in their decision to get the shot or not.

A study of data from the Pfizer and Moderna clinical trials by Dr. Peter Doshi and colleagues provides additional insight on these issues. First, Doshi et al found: "The excess risk of serious adverse events of special interest surpassed the risk reduction for COVID-19 hospitalization relative to the placebo group in both Pfizer and Moderna trials (2.3 and 6.4 per 10,000 participants, respectively)." [407]

As discussed in Part 1 concerning Pfizer's risk reduction calculations, Doshi also noted that the number of confirmed cases used by Pfizer to calculate the risk reduction rates (a total of 170) "were dwarfed by a category of disease called 'suspected covid-19'—those with symptomatic covid-19 that were not PCR confirmed." If those 3,410 suspected-but-not-confirmed cases had been included in the calculations, Doshi estimated the RRR would have been only between 19% to 29% instead of 95%, far below the FDA's minimum of 50%.[408] *Could it be that Pfizer was manipulating how many in the suspected or symptomatic group they would actually test in order to come up with an RRR of 95%?*

CLINICAL TRIAL DATA SHOW A DECLINE IN HEALTH

Dr. J. Bart Classen, MD, is an immunologist and former NIH scientist. He is one of many who have analyzed the clinical trial data of Pfizer, Moderna and Johnson & Johnson. He begins by noting: "For decades, **true scientists have warned that pivotal clinical trial designs for vaccines are dangerously flawed and outdated.**"[409] Such was the case with the COVID-19 trials. For one thing, he said: "Reductions in infection rates, hospitalization rates and even death with COVID-19 are poor surrogate markers for health and are not proper primary endpoints for a vaccine clinical trial." Classen also stated:

> "Results prove that none of the vaccines provide a health benefit and all pivotal trials show a statically (*sic*) [statistically] significant increase in "all cause severe morbidity" in the vaccinated group compared to the placebo group."

Among his other conclusions, Classen also states:

> "...in fact, all the vaccines cause a decline in health in the immunized groups...
>
> "... reducing severe COVID-19 infections does not equate to enhanced survival especially when the vaccine can cause clotting, heart disease and many other severe adverse events. Potential vaccine recipients need to know if the vaccine improves their survival in order for them to make an informed consent to be immunized. Unfortunately, the current studies with COVID-19 vaccines in fact show they cause a decline in health.
>
> "The actual health decline caused by the vaccines is probably much worse than what is depicted in Table 1 for many reasons."

The "Table 1" referred to is entitled "All Cause Severe Morbidity," found in his study. It reflects combined data from the Pfizer, Moderna and Johnson & Johnson trials upon which his comments are based.

Dr. Classen had even more critical remarks about the trials and the manufacturers' conduct:

> "Regrettably, the vaccines did not reduce morbidity but caused an increase in severe events. Worse, the pivotal clinical trials were never designed to show a benefit in 'all-cause mortality' or reduction 'in all cause severe morbidity.' The fact that the trials were never designed to show these health benefits is an admission

that those developing the vaccines never expected the vaccines to result in measurable health benefits."

He concluded his study by stating: "Mass immunization with COVID-19 vaccines is certainly leading to a catastrophic public health event."

Another analysis of the shortcomings of the Pfizer trials and how they actually demonstrated a decline in health and a risk-benefit ratio that did not support its vaccine was prepared by the Canadian COVID Care Alliance (CCCA), a consortium of more than 500 doctors, based on Pfizer's 6-month data released on September 15, 2021.[410] The CCA's analysis is presented in a video entitled "The Pfizer Inoculations for COVID-19: More Harm Than Good." [411] The CCCA noted that while Pfizer's own data showed a 91.5% efficacy rate in preventing COVID infection, its other data showed that it came at the expense of an increase in other more serious illness and deaths. The CCCA also noted that this data was not in the main report itself, but can only be found by digging into the supplementary appendix.[412] See Table 17.

Table 17.[413] Analysis by Canadian COVID Care Alliance from the Pfizer 6-Month Report showing comparison of efficacy and adverse event results for the treatment and placebo groups.

Pfizer 6-Month Report Data	BNT162b2 (Pfizer vax)	Placebo	Risk Change
Efficacy (Meaning # of people diagnosed with COVID-19)	77	850	-91%
Related Adverse Event (Meaning an investigator has assessed it as related to the BNT162b2 injection)	5,241	1,311	+300%
Any Serious Adverse Event (Interferes significantly with normal function)	262	150	+75%
Any Serious Adverse Event (Involves visit to ER or hospitalization)	127	116	+10%

Other Major Wrongdoing Pervades Clinical Trials. Others have analyzed the many shortcomings of the COVID vaccine clinical trials, as well as the clinical trial process in general. Dr. James Thorp and Dr. Deborah Viglione, as well as others, also point out that there should have been randomized, double-blinded placebo-controlled clinical trials before these shots were ever released to the general public. Sasha Latypova has also analyzed documents related to the clinical trials. In one article, she discusses various "deficiencies, omission, and gaps, which were very obvious but were never questioned by the regulators or health authorities." She pointed to the lack of safety studies which were either standard or mandatory and the "scientific dishonesty in those studies which were performed are so obvious and glaring that they cannot be attributed to the incompetence of the manufacturers and regulators." [414] She points to a "complete breakdown of the regular process of drug development and approval."

An article posted in *Technocracy News* reveals that "Not recording injuries, or recording them improperly, are a common tactic used to fudge results and make a vaccine appear safer than it is. Another common strategy is to exclude any parameter that turns out to be problematic, and that includes participants who are injured." [415] The article then cites that particular problem with respect to Pfizer's pediatric COVID trial where about 3,000 of the 4,526 children who were enrolled were excluded from their final calculations, but no explanation was given as to why. That was described as a "huge red flag," a sentiment echoed by Dr. Claire Craig, as reported in Part 2. *If a significant percentage of the 3,000 had suffered a fairly serious adverse reaction, think of how that would skew their trial results which should have then led to a denial of the EUA for that age group.*

An article entitled "How Vaccine Trials Routinely Rig the Results," published July 8, 2022, provides an analysis by Dr. Joseph Mercola of the overall problem of how clinical trials can be manipulated.[416] An article on the *Chemical Violence* website made the following comment about the Future Framework discussed above: "While many examples of rigged vaccine trials had been recorded over the years, the future framework served as an extreme expansion and formalization of the scheme." [417] *Is it only a matter of time before the FDA does away with all clinical trials for all future new drugs?*

[407] Fraiman, Joseph and Erviti, Juan and Jones, Mark and Greenland, Sander and Whelan, Patrick and Kaplan, Robert M. and Doshi, Peter, Serious Adverse Events of Special Interest Following mRNA Vaccination in Randomized Trials. Available at SSRN: https://ssrn.com/abstract=4125239

[408] https://www.fda.gov/media/144245/download, p. 52

[409] J. Bart Classen, MD, "US COVID-19 Vaccines Proven to Cause More Harm than Good Based on Pivotal Clinical Trial Data Analyzed Using the Proper Scientific Endpoint, "All Cause Severe Morbidity". Trends Int Med, 2021, Vol 1, Issue 1. https://www.scivisionpub.com/pdfs/us-covid19-vaccines-proven-to-cause-more-harm-than-good-based-on-pivotal-clinical-trial-data-analyzed-using-the-proper-scientific--1811.pdf (report issued July 24, 2021, accepted August 25, 2021)

[410] Thomas SJ, Moreira ED Jr, Kitchin N, et al. Safety and efficacy of the BNT162b2 mRNA Covid-19 vaccine through 6 months. N Engl J Med 2021;385:1761-73. DOI: 10.1056/NEJMoa2110345; https://www.nejm.org/doi/full/10.1056/NEJMoa2110345

[411] http://www.preearth.net/videos/clinical-proof-pfizer-shots-do-more-harm-than-good.mp4

[412] Supplement to: Thomas SJ, Moreira ED Jr, Kitchin N, et al. Safety and efficacy of the BNT162b2 mRNA Covid-19 vaccine through 6 months. N Engl J Med2021;385:1761-73. DOI: 10.1056/NEJMoa2110345; https://www.nejm.org/doi/suppl/10.1056/NEJMoa2110345/suppl_file/nejmoa2110345_appendix.pdf

[413] https://www.canadiancovidcarealliance.org/wp-content/uploads/2021/12/The-COVID-19-Inoculations-More-Harm-Than-Good-REV-Dec-16-2021.pdf, p. 11

[414] Sasha Latypova, https://www.trialsitenews.com/a/did-pfizer-perform-adequate-preclinical-safety-studies-for-bnt162b2-cf0c7fc4 (June 28, 2022)

[415] Dr. Joseph Mercola, https://www.technocracy.news/bio-security-state-big-pharmas-complete-takeover-of-fda/ (July 8, 2022)

[416] https://media.mercola.com/ImageServer/Public/2022/July/PDF/covid-19-vaccine-trials-results-pdf.pdf

[417] Mary Villareal, https://www.chemicalviolence.com/2022-07-14-fda-future-framework-allows-bypass-vaccine-testing.html (July 14, 2022)

Chapter 29
Natural Immunity is Superior to Vaccine Immunity

Many studies show that natural immunity is superior to any vaccine immunity. That was the conclusion of a study from Israel reported in December 2021.[418] It showed that those with natural immunity had an infection rate of only 10.5 per 100,000 four to six months following their recovery, as compared with a rate of 69.2 per 100,000 among the vaccinated. That is a rate of more than *6X or 600%* higher among the vaccinated.

In addition, the number of severe cases among those with natural immunity was only 0.5% of all cases, compared with 0.9% among the vaccinated, almost twice as many. That article also stated that:

> "The naturally immune, though, are better protected against both infection and severe disease, according to a large body of research that includes the latest study from Israel."

The article then quotes Dr. Paul Alexander, an epidemiologist with the Early COVID Care Experts who has collected 141 studies on natural immunity. Of those who had recovered from COVID, he said:

> "...all the data that we're looking at will suggest that you have bulletproof natural immunity, which is much more robust and comprehensive than vaccine immunity."

A recent study in Qatar that focused on long-term natural immunity in unvaccinated people found that natural immunity was 97.3% effective "against severe, critical or fatal COVID-19 reinfection, and with no evidence of waning." [419] Similar results were also reported for those 50 years and older. Therefore, they concluded that natural immunity was superior to vaccine immunity, such as revealed in a recent Swedish study cited by the Qatar group which found in May 2022 that two doses of COVID-19 were only 54% effective against the Omicron variant. That barely passes the FDA's threshold of 50% efficacy.

Johns Hopkins surgeon and professor Dr. Marty Makary confirmed in July 2022 that over 200 formal studies found that natural immunity was superior to vaccine immunity. He added that unvaccinated people "pose no public health threat now that population immunity is high." [420] In fact, Dr. Michael Yeadon says that if these shots were really about public health, one group of people you would *not* vaccinate are those who have recovered from COVID. It actually makes them *worse* off.[421] ***Why are those with natural immunity being encouraged or forced to get the shots? Why is the science NOT being followed?***

---

[418] Zachary Stieber, https://www.theepochtimes.com/natural-immunity-more-protective-over-time-than-covid-19-vaccination-study_4149953.html (Dec. 13, 2021)

[419] Zachary Stieber, https://www.theepochtimes.com/natural-immunity-97-percent-effective-against-severe-covid-19-after-14-months-study_4586731.html (July 9, 2022, updated July 11, 2022)

[420] Emily Miller, https://www.theepochtimes.com/exclusive-large-texas-hospital-faces-staff-shortages-despite-covid-19-vaccine-mandate_4602092.html (July 18, 2022)

[421] Dr. Michael Yeadon presentation, https://odysee.com/@Quasar:3/Mike-Yeadon-Testimony-for-the-Grand-Jury:9 (testimony date Feb. 4, 2022)

Chapter 30
Reports From Autopsies, the Funeral Industry & Life Insurance Companies

Autopsy Data

Dr. Peter Schirmacher, Chief Pathologist at the University of Heidelberg and Acting Chairman of the German Society of Pathology, is considered by *The Pathologist* to be one of the top 100 pathologists in the world. He did autopsies on 40 people who died within 14 days of a COVID shot. He concluded that 30-40% of them died *from* the vaccine, and in his opinion, the frequency of fatal consequences of vaccinations is "underestimated."[422] Therefore, his 30-40% figures could be much higher.

Other autopsies performed by two other experienced pathologists, Dr. Arne Burkhardt and Prof. Dr, Walter Lang, showed results consistent with Dr. Schirmacher's findings. They did autopsies on ten people who had recently been vaccinated. Despite the small sample, they found three rare autoimmune diseases, but the most alarming finding was that *"The lymphocytes are running amok in all organs,"* according to Prof. Lang. "We're missing out on 90 percent," he said, of the number of fatal vaccine reactions.[423] All three pathologists have called for more autopsies on recently vaccinated deceased persons. **But Anthony Fauci has discouraged autopsies in the U.S. – why do you suppose that is?**

Drs. Sucharit Bhakdi and Arne Burkhardt did presentations at a Doctors for COVID Ethics Symposium on December 10, 2021.[424] They had done autopsies on 15 patients who died from 7 days to 6 months after vaccination. Significantly, the coroner had decided that none of these deaths were caused by the vaccine. However, the two doctors found "in 14 of the 15 patients there was widespread evidence of the body attacking itself, something that is never seen before. The heart was attacked in all 14 cases." A summary of their findings and *why COVID vaccines cannot work* is found in an article cited in the endnote below.

Pathologists, other doctors and medical examiners: might you be overlooking something in determining the cause of death of vaccinated persons?

Dr. Ryan Cole, MD, is a board certified anatomic and clinical pathologist who trained at the Mayo Clinic. He runs a large independent lab and is probably in the top ten of American pathologists in terms of the number of patients he has seen in his career.[425] In an interview, he explained that there is a simple test that can be done during post-mortem exams that reveals whether or not the death was caused by the COVID shots, but these tests are not being done.[426] He added that *the standard pathological slide stains that are run during these exams do not show this, and that is one reason why the vaccine's causative role in death is not being found.* The other reason doctors are not finding the vaccine connection is simply that they are not looking for it. Cole recommends the protocol developed by Dr. Arne Burkhardt which uses special stains that detect the spike protein.[427] Cole has made some additions to that protocol which he provided to Steve Kirsch.[428] Burkhardt says they were able to successfully detect it "using an antibody specific for the spike protein by conventional immunohistochemistry."[429]

The only doctors Cole knows of who are doing this test are seven doctors in Germany (including Burkhardt) and perhaps one other in the United States, besides himself. One other very important point he made was that this test can be run even a long time after death, if the tissue samples were preserved. That may help grieving family members who still want to know even a year or more later if the death of their loved one was vaccine-related.

Reports from Embalmers/Funeral Directors/Casket Manufacturers

Not surprisingly, funeral directors and embalmers have also been reporting unprecedented findings about deceased vaccinated persons. A funeral director in the UK says he "has never seen as many deaths" (since the vaccines) and is reporting about a 500-600% increase in the number of deaths among young adults. They had all been vaccinated.[430]

The report of the Canadian casket manufacturer who was quoted in Parts 1 and 2 is also relevant here.[431] His comment that their business actually declined about 60% during 2020 stands in sharp contrast to what happened after the vaccine rollout in late 2020, through 2021 and into

2022. Not only did the increase in casket sales become "staggering," but his comments about the huge increase of selling 5 years' worth of child caskets in 7 months was particularly troubling.

An American Certified Embalmer, Richard Hirschman, has been embalming for over 20 years. He reports seeing veins and arteries filled with rubbery clots and strange fibrous materials that were completely filling the vascular system in the bodies of deceased vaxxed persons. He had never seen this phenomenon before, which has created challenges in the embalming process.[432] Even his colleagues who have been embalming for 30-50 years are observing the same things that they had never seen before either. These have been described as "white fibrous clots," "synthetic tissue," or "rubbery substances."[433]

Hirschman also said that January 2021 – right after the vaccine rollout – was the busiest he had ever been. He started keeping track in November 2021 of how many people he is seeing these strange "things" in. In January 2022, out of 35 people he embalmed, this condition was present in 20-24 of them. He said: "If this is caused by the vaccine, can you imagine how many people will be dying from this? Because people can't live with this kind of substance floating around in their vessels."

Another embalmer, Cary Watkins, has had over 50 years of embalming experience and has known Hirschman for many years. He vouched for Hirschman's credibility and his excellence as an embalmer. He also confirmed that he has seen the same types of unusual clots Hirschman has reported.[434] *The Epoch Times* has also confirmed, after Hirschman was the first embalmer to come forward, that several other embalmers from different states have reported seeing the same kind of fibrous and rubbery clot-like substances described by Hirschman. They did not know if these were caused by COVID-19, the vaccines or other causes.[435] *The Epoch Times* article also quoted Hirschman as saying: "They're not even dead from COVID. They're dying of sudden heart attacks, strokes, cancers. It doesn't seem to matter what these people die of nowadays, so many of them have the same anomalies in their blood."

UK funeral director John O'Looney has also been speaking out very passionately about what he has seen in his industry since COVID began. Dozens of other funeral directors in the UK share his experience. He noted that 2020 was actually quieter than 2019 in the funeral business even with all the deaths in 2020 attributed to COVID (but were not actually COVID). They only started seeing "pandemic level deaths" after the vaccines started. He has seen the same kinds of white, fibrous clot-like substances as Hirschman. By the end of 2021, he had seen more people under 40 die in just the first 12 months after the vaccine rollout than in the prior 10 years. He continues to see more and more deaths among people of all ages. [436]

Figures 1 – 3 below are photos of just a few of the samples presented by Hirschman showing different kinds of rubbery, fibrous clot-like substances that he and other embalmers are finding in the vascular system of deceased vaccinated persons. These unusual substances are not like typical blood clots, which easily fall apart when picked up, according to Hirschman.[437] Photos of other types of samples, as well as more detail of his findings, can be found in various interviews he has done in the independent media.[438]

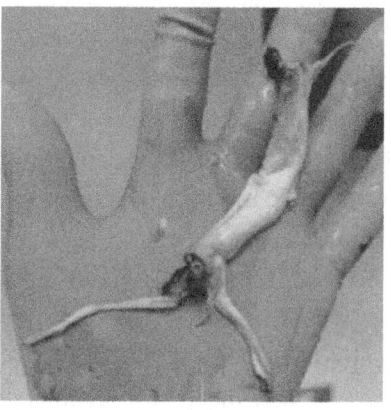

Figure 1 (on right) : [439] This is a large white, fibrous, rubbery "clot" from the vascular system of a deceased vaccinated person.

Figure 2 (below): [440] This is a close-up example of several smaller clot-like strings from the vascular system of one deceased vaccinated person.

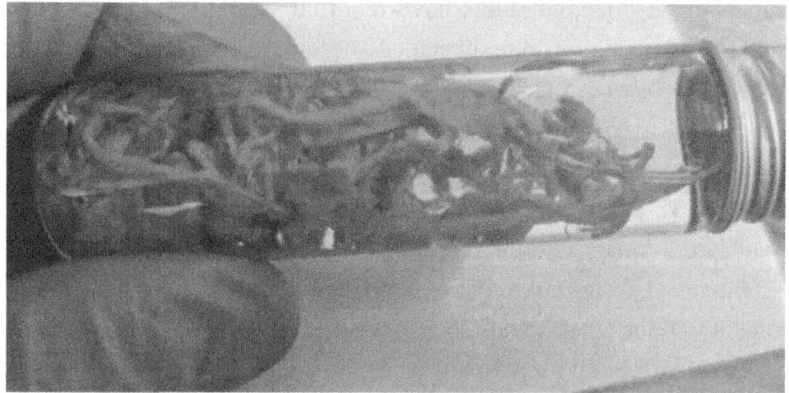

Figure 3:[441] The contents of the 7 vials below are from the vascular systems of 7 different deceased vaccinated persons.

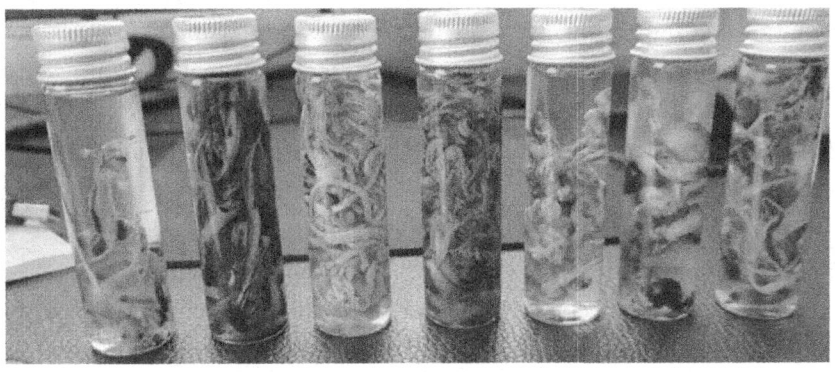

More recently, Hirschman said that he had started finding similar substances in the bodies of deceased *unvaxxed* persons as well. However, he found out that those people had all received blood transfusions. That obviously raises a serious concern about the safety of local blood supplies.[442]

Data from Life Insurance Company Claims

Another reliable source of data that reveals the extent of impacts from the vaccines is life insurance claims. One America is a $100 billion national life insurance company. Its CEO Scott Davidson reported at the end of 2021 that in the 3rd quarter of 2021, deaths among working age people aged 18-64 years old had skyrocketed by 40% over pre-pandemic levels. In fact, he said:

> "'We are seeing, right now, the highest death rates we have seen in the history of this business – not just at OneAmerica ...The data is consistent across every player in that business. ...
>
> "'And what we saw just in third quarter, we're seeing it continue into fourth quarter, is that death rates are up 40% over what they were pre-pandemic....
>
> "'Just to give you an idea of how bad that is, a three-sigma or a one-in-200-year catastrophe would be a 10% increase over pre-pandemic... *So 40% is just unheard of.*'" [443]

Davidson also noted: "What the data is showing to us is that the deaths that are being reported as COVID deaths greatly understate the actual death losses among working-age people from the pandemic. It may not all be COVID on their death certificate, but deaths are up just huge, huge numbers."

Davidson also said that it is not just the death rate that is significantly higher. There has also been an 'uptick" in the number of disability claims. He said at first the increase was for short-term disability, but later they were more for long-term disabilities. He expected the cost of disability claims to be more than $100 million, just for his company.

It appears that at least at that time, Davidson and other life insurance executives had not yet connected the large increase in deaths and long-term disabilities to the vaccines. *Could this be largely because many doctors are not indicating any connection to the vaccines on the death certificates?*

The same article in January 2022 that quoted Davidson's data also reports information from Brian Tabor, the president of the Indiana Hospital Association. Tabor said that hospitals in Indiana at that time were being flooded with patients "with many different conditions," and the number of hospitalizations was higher than before the vaccines were rolled out. In fact, he said, it is the highest in 5 years. He added that only 37% of the of ICU beds were taken up by COVID-19 patients, so the vast majority of patients are there for other reasons. *How many might be there because of vaccine injuries?*

Dr. Robert Malone had damning words to say about the implications of the One America data:[444]

> "AT A MINIMUM, based on my reading, one has to conclude that if this report holds and is confirmed by others in the dry world of life insurance actuaries, we have both a huge human tragedy and a profound public policy failure of the US Government and US HHS....
>
> "IF this holds true, then the genetic vaccines so aggressively promoted have failed, and the clear federal campaign to prevent early treatment with lifesaving drugs has contributed to a massive, avoidable loss of life."
>
> "AT WORST, this report implies that the federal workplace vaccine mandates have driven what appear to be a true crime against humanity …"

Aegon, a Dutch company that does two-thirds of its business in the Americas, reported that claims here went from $31 million in 3rd quarter 2020 up to $111 million in 3rd quarter 2021.[445] Also significant is the statement by Aegon's CEO that: "Performance improvements across most of our businesses ... were offset by elevated mortality in the United States."

In June 2022, it was reported that Lincoln National, the 5th largest life insurance company in the U.S., reported "a 163% increase in death benefits paid out under its group insurance policies, in 2021 compared to 2020."[446] In contrast, the increase in 2020, the pre-vax COVID year, over 2019 was only 9%. That report also said that "Prudential and Northwestern Mutual also show significant increases — increases much larger in 2021 than in 2020, indicating that the cure was worse than the disease — much worse."

Edward Dowd is a former Wall Street executive and successful portfolio manager for BlackRock, one of the leading providers of investment, advisory and risk management solutions. He and a Wall Street insurance expert analyzed CDC data for the Millennial generation for the period March 2021-February 2022. Their results: this 25 to 44-year-old group suffered **more than 61,000 excess deaths** during that period, representing an **84% increase.** They noted a "particularly significant 'spike' in mortality in the fall of 2021 ... that cannot be explained by the delta variant, opioids, suicides or other causes."[447]

Dowd said that was the **highest increase in excess deaths of any age group** in 2021 – even seven times higher than the Silent Generation (those who are older than 85). He has also said that there were **100,000 excess deaths** for the same period posted among the Gen X'ers, ages 45-64.[448] "'The thing to remember about the insurance industry," he said, "is that they make money by predicting health-care issues and death-rate issues – and they do that fairly accurately, and with precision. So any disruption to that upsets their business model,' he said. 'And this is a big disruption.'"[449]

He also has said that he had been contacted by a "very high senior chief risk officer actuary out of a major insurance company who wants to compare notes." [450] So the word is getting out, and his friends on Wall Street are listening.[451] In August 2022, Dowd reported that his data had been confirmed by the Society of Actuaries Research Institute.[452] He said that their data showed a 100% increase for the 35-44 year old group during the 3rd quarter 2021, and that first quarter numbers for 2022 were also showing about a 20% increase in excess deaths, which was carrying over into the second quarter as well.

Shortly after his initial revelations in early 2022, on April 29 Dowd posted on his GETTR social media page the conclusion he had come to after analyzing the data, that **"the largest fraud ever is embodied in this simple phrase: 'Safe & Effective.'"**

---

[422] TLB Staff, https://www.thelibertybeacon.com/jab-is-cause-of-death-in-30-40-of-recently-vaccinated-german-chief-pathologist/ (Sept 15, 2021)

[423] Professors Arne Burkhardt and Walter Lang, https://principia-scientific.com/pathologists-shocking-finding-from-deaths-after-covid-19-jabs/ (Sept. 27, 2021)

[424] Dr.Sucharit Bhakdi and Dr. Arne Burkhardt,. Summary: "On COVID vaccines: why they cannot work, and irrefutable evidence of their causative role in deaths after vaccination," https://www.bitchute.com/video/fHIT55iM4Zv9/ (Dec. 24, 2021); written report at: https://doctors4covidethics.org/wp-content/uploads/2021/12/end-covax.pdf (Dec. 10, 2021)

[425] Steve Kirsch, https://stevekirsch.substack.com/p/my-interviews-with-ryan-cole-deb (Aug,13, 2022)

[426] Id.

[427] https://www.skirsch.com/covid/Burkhardt.pdf

[428] Steve Kirsch, https://stevekirsch.substack.com/p/my-interviews-with-ryan-cole-deb (Aug. 13, 2022)

[429] https://pathologie-konferenz.de/en/ (Jan. 17, 2022)

[430] Jim Hoft, https://www.thegatewaypundit.com/2022/01/never-seen-many-deaths-around-500-600-increase-funeral-director-uk-reveals-increasing-number-death-vaccinated-young-adults/ (Jan. 28, 2022)

[431] Miranda Sellick, https://rairfoundation.com/coffins-for-children-ordered-in-bulk-first-time-in-over-30-years-exclusive-interview/ (July 14, 2022)

[432] Dr. Jane Ruby, https://www.redvoicemedia.com/2022/01/worldwide-exclusive-embalmers-find-veins-arteries-filled-with-never-before-seen-rubbery-clots/ (Jan. 28, 2022)

[433] Rhoda Wilson, https://expose-news.com/2022/06/28/scaffold-tissue-and-nanowires-most-likely-cause-sads/ (June 28, 2022)

[434] Steve Kirsch phone interview with Cary Watkins, https://rumble.com/vuycmg-embalmer-with-50-years-of-experience-verifies-hirschmans-story.html (Feb. 14, 2022)

[435] Enrico Rigoso, https://www.theepochtimes.com/embalmers-have-been-finding-numerous-long-fibrous-clots-that-lack-post-mortem-characteristics_4696015.html?utm_source=ref_share&utm_campaign=tw&rs=SHRNRRCV (Sept. 2, 2022)

[436] https://stopworldcontrol.com/director/; see also John O'Looney interviewed by Laura Lynn Tyler Thompson, https://rumble.com/v1hhebv-live-with-john-oloone.html (August 26, 2022), and

https://www.globalresearch.ca/video-funeral-director-john-olooney-talks-about-his-recent-clients/5764137 (Dec. 29, 2021)

[437] Kevin Hughes, https://citizens.news/639893.html (July 22, 2022)

[438] Richard Hirschman interviewed on Infowars, https://www.redvoicemedia.com/video/2022/06/must-see-mortician-finds-massive-hand-sized-clots-in-cadavers-after-vax-video/ (June 14, 2022); also, Kevin Hughes, https://citizens.news/639893.html (July 22, 2022)

[439] Courtesy of Richard Hirschman. See also Hirschman interview on Infowars (above)

[440] Id.

[441] Courtesy of Richard Hirschman. See also Enrico Rigoso, Sept. 2, 2022 article

[442] Richard Hirschman, interviewed by Maria Zeee, https://www.redvoicemedia.com/2022/07/warning-extremely-graphic-structures-killing-injected-1-year-after-shot-whistleblower-richard-hirschman-with-maria-zeee/ (July 19, 2022)

[443] Margaret Menge, https://www.thecentersquare.com/indiana/indiana-life-insurance-ceo-says-deaths-are-up-40-among-people-ages-18-64/article_71473b12-6b1e-11ec-8641-5b2c06725e2c.html (Jan. 1, 2022)

[444] Dr. Robert Malone, "What if the largest experiment on human beings in history is a failure?" https://rwmalonemd.substack.com/p/what-if-the-largest-experiment-on (Jan. 2, 2022)

[445] Toby Sterling, https://www.reuters.com/business/finance/aegon-q3-operating-result-down-16-us-covid-linked-claims-2021-11-11/ (Nov. 11, 2021)

[446] https://expose-news.com/2022/06/23/life-insurance-176percent-increase-payouts-deaths-2021/ (June 23, 2022)

[447] Art Moore, https://www.wnd.com/2022/03/wall-street-analyst-covid-vaccines-greatest-fraud-history/ (March 16, 2022)

[448] Alexandra Bruce, https://www.lewrockwell.com/2022/03/no_author/edward-dowd-on-future-recession-shocking-findings-in-the-cdc-covid-data-and-democide/ (March 12, 2022) (from Dowd's GETTR account)

[449] Art Moore, https://www.wnd.com/2022/03/wall-street-analyst-covid-vaccines-greatest-fraud-history/ (March 16, 2022)

[450] Edward Dowd interview, https://www.bitchute.com/video/fCvcEypV0Ncd/ (posted March 27, 2022)

[451] Edward Dowd comments at 2022 Maui Earth Day Festival, May 2, 2022, https://rumble.com/v13c6f0-the-greatest-fraud-in-history-ed-dowd-at-maui-earth-day-5122.html

[452] Edward Dowd interviewed by Steve Bannon, https://rumble.com/v1gocc1-edward-dowd-new-actuarial-report-reaffirms-trail-of-death-caused-by-vaccine.html (Aug. 2022)

Chapter 31
Other Evidence of Adverse Impacts:
D-dimer Tests, the Story That Backfired, & Who Needs to Be Protected From Whom?

D-dimer testing

Canadian Dr. Charles Hoffe has reported that D-dimer testing he did on patients who received the mRNA COVID shots revealed elevated D-dimer levels. He reported that 62% were already showing microscopic blood clots.[453] Dr. Hoffe went public with his information in the spring of 2021. After doing so, the Interior Health Authority (Canada) suspended his clinical privileges. He was accused of causing "vaccine-hesitancy." Because of his suspension, he was not allowed to continue working in the emergency room at the hospital in his community. He has continued speaking out about the dangers of the COVID vaccines, stating that *"what we have seen in the last 18 months since the start of this vaccine rollout is the biggest disaster in medical history. Never before in medical history has any medical treatment killed and maimed so many people."*[454]

The Survey That Backfired.

On September 10, 2021, ABC affiliate station WXYZ in Detroit made a post on its Facebook page asking readers to contact the station if they had a story they would be willing to share about a loved one who had not been vaccinated and died of COVID. The station was working on a story on the subject and was looking for people's stories to support their premise.

It is reported that within just a few days, there were already 39,000 comments. As of January 28, 2022, there were 261,000 comments and it had been shared 217,000 times. At some point the comments were turned off. However, very few of those comments were what the station expected or asked for. Instead, they got *thousands of posts about loved ones who died shortly after getting the COVID vaccines or had adverse reactions to the shots.*[455] Several posts were asking the station: *when are you going to do that story, about sad stories of those who got the shots and died or suffered injuries?* Many people commented on how the station's post had backfired. Others who read a lot of the posts also reported not seeing any about unvaxxed people dying of COVID.

Even though this is anecdotal evidence, and many posts were about the backfiring and expressions of sympathy for those reporting losses of loved ones, it is still significant evidence of the extent of the problem and the devastation these shots are causing. It is very heart-breaking to read their stories. One after another after another of people whose loved ones either died or experienced a serious adverse reaction within minutes, hours or days of getting the shots. And most of them were relatively healthy working-age people.

Who Needs to Be Protected From Whom?

The official narrative is that the "unvaccinated are a threat to the vaccinated." According to Anthony Fauci, as of August 2021: "As we've said all along this is fundamentally a pandemic among the unvaccinated...That is proven true."[456] Besides the fact that the above data "disprove" that assertion, if there was ever a "pandemic of the unvaccinated," it is only because the CDC changed the definition of "unvaccinated" to include untold thousands of people who had received at least one shot! For that, the unvaxxed have been shamed, discriminated against, called unpatriotic, and much worse. In some places, they are barred from entering certain businesses due to authoritarian "vaccination passport" requirements.

Where is the logic in that? Is it not it an admission that the shots are NOT really so effective? If they were effective, why should the vaxxed have anything to fear from the unvaxxed? **It makes no sense**. Actually, with regard to these shots, the evidence shows that it is the unvaxxed who have reasons to be concerned about the vaxxed, instead of the other way around.

Shedding/Transmission. Shedding has to do with vaxxed persons causing symptoms in unvaxxed through close contact. Some say the correct term is "transmission," because shedding is a "virus term." Regardless, the concept is the same. As explained in a briefing by America's Frontline Doctors, a consortium of hundreds of doctors who have been successfully treating COVID-19 patients with their protocols:

"shedding appears to be causing wide variety of autoimmune disease (where the body attacks its own tissue) in some persons. Worldwide cases of pericarditis, shingles, pneumonia, blood clots in the extremities and brain, Bell's Palsy, vaginal bleeding and miscarriages have been reported in persons who are near persons who have been vaccinated." [457]

One of the most common shedding problems relates to a female's monthly cycle, according to Dr. Lee Merritt, MD, a former military doctor who was also an orthopaedic and spinal surgeon for many years.[458] Dr. Christiane Northrup, a board-certified Ob-Gyn physician who has been a leader in the field of women's health and wellness for many years, explains that even in 2021, "thousands upon thousands of unvaccinated women ... are experiencing dramatic changes" in their monthly cycles from being around women who had received the COVID shots.[459] Shedding has disrupted the cycles of unvaxxed women of child-bearing age and even caused post-menopausal women to have bleeding problems after coming into contact with a vaxxed person. Noting that "something is clearly being transmitted," Dr. Northrup has told of "horrific stories" about babies just a few months old having blood clots coming out of their bodies after having contact with people who had recently received COVID shots.[460]

Dr. Merritt also cites and explains highlights of a 2015 paper written by the FDA entitled "Design and Analysis of Shedding Studies for Virus or Bacteria-Based Gene Therapy and Oncolytic Products — Guidance for Industry." [461] That means the FDA has been aware of this problem at least since 2015. *Did they warn the public or the medical community about it?* **Doctors, are many of your female patients, both those of reproductive age and even post-menopausal women, complaining of such problems?** Dr. Simone Gold, the founder of AFLDS, has also pointed to a Pfizer document in which she says Pfizer "'acknowledges this mechanism' of this shedding" during its trial period.[462]

Another statement in the AFLDS briefing expresses concern "that some children will become COVID symptomatic after their parents and teachers get vaccinated." In fact, Dr. Philippe VanWelbergen, a UK physician and scientist explained in an interview that he believes this is happening.[463] He specializes in biomedicine and regularly runs red blood cell morphology tests on his patients. He is now finding that the blood

OTHER EVIDENCE OF ADVERSE IMPACTS

samples of some of his unvaxxed patients, including young children, are showing the same kind of blood damage he was originally seeing (after the vaccine rollout) only in vaccinated patients. He believes this has occurred through transmission by close contact with vaxxed persons. In one case, he says, the child's parents had not received the shots either. During that interview he showed photos of the damaged red blood cells. *Where are the warnings from the government or manufacturers?*

Dangers of Vaccinated Pilots, Drivers and Others. Another reason that everyone has cause to be concerned is the danger posed by vaxxed pilots or drivers on the roads. Steve Kirsch, founder of the Vaccine Safety Research Foundation, cites data from the Oct/Nov 2021 issue of the ALPA (Air Line Pilot Association) magazine which showed that 111 commercial airline pilots died in the first 9 months of 2021 – compared with only 6 pilots who died in 2020, and only 1 in 2019.[464]

There has been at least one report of a pilot death in mid-flight shortly after getting his second COVID shot. Fortunately, because commercial passenger flights require more than one pilot, the co-pilot was able to successfully land the plane.[465] The airline claimed the report was false.[466]

American Airlines pilot Captain Robert Snow suffered cardiac arrest in the cockpit just a few minutes after landing and pulling up to the gate.[467] If that heart event had happened while still in the process of landing or in the air, it could have ended in disaster. Even though he miraculously survived to tell about what happened, it was a career-ending event. He attributes his heart problem to the vaccine that he was forced to take to keep his job. He also said: "'There was absolutely no warning preceding my collapse in the cockpit. It was literally as if someone 'pulled the plug.'"[468]

Pilot Josh Yoder is the co-founder of the group U.S. Freedom Flyers. In the same article about Capt. Snow, Yoder told interviewer Steve Kirsch that many other commercial pilots were calling him. They were saying that they, too, were suffering from heart problems after getting a COVID injection required by their employer. However, they were afraid to say anything out of fear of losing their job.

Another frightening report was given by a former commercial airline captain about the significant increase in emergency alerts by pilots.[469] He said that typically he would get alerts only 1 to 4 times per month. But over the last couple of months (early 2022) (after pilots were pressured or forced to get the "vaccines"), he said that sometimes he has been getting up to 10 alerts per day. Hopefully that situation has improved considerably since the time of that report in early spring of 2022.

How long will vaxxed pilots be able to pass their required check-ups? This is not only a threat to the pilots, passengers and people on the ground, but also to the whole airline industry.

What might happen if the sole pilot of a smaller aircraft suffers a blood clot or heart event during flight? Or what about a cognitive issue that affects the mental clarity needed to safely fly and land the plane? Cody Flint was the sole pilot on a smaller non-passenger plane when he suddenly experienced a serious adverse reaction to a COVID vaccine in mid-air that could have ended in tragedy.[470] It is a miracle he was able to land safely. He does not even know how he managed to land the plane.[471] The article cited in the reference tells his story and that of several others that are simply heart-breaking accounts of career-ending injuries due to vaccine mandates.

Have you noticed how many thousands of flights have been cancelled in recent months? It was not just the pilots who were subject to the mandates, but also the other support personnel like baggage handlers and maintenance crews as well as flight attendants.

Drivers. Given how so many vaxxed people experience sudden death or impairment shortly after the shots, and the unknown long-term effects, this presents potential safety concerns for all drivers.

And what about surgeons? What if a surgeon in the middle of a surgery suddenly collapses or has a cognitive impairment that causes serious harm to a patient? There are other professions as well whose work may present a hazard to others if they were to experience a sudden problem as a result of the vaccine.

---

[453] https://covidcalltohumanity.org/2021/09/08/dr-charles-hoffe-mrna-vaccines-will-kill-most-people-through-heart-failure-62-already-have-microscopic-blood-clots/ (Sept. 8, 2021)

[454] Dr. Charles Hoffe, speaking at a rally in Vancouver, BC, Canada, https://www.thetruthseeker.co.uk/?p=257546 (Aug. 19, 2022)

[455] https://luis46pr.wordpress.com/2021/09/17/local-detroit-tv-asks-for-stories-of-unvaxxed-dying-from-covid-gets-over-180k-responses-of-vaccine-injured-and-dead-instead/ (Sept. 17, 2021)

[456] Connor Perrett, https://www.businessinsider.com/fauci-unvaccinated-could-lead-to-variant-worse-than-delta-2021-8 (Aug. 8, 2021)

OTHER EVIDENCE OF ADVERSE IMPACTS

[457] https://americasfrontlinedoctors.org/2/action_alerts/identifying-post-vaccination-complications-their-causes-an-analysis-of-covid-19-patient-data/

[458] Dr. Lee D. Merritt, "COVID-19 Vaccines: A "Cure" Worse Than the Disease?" https://thenewamerican.com/magazine/tna3713/page/130713 (July 5, 2021)

[459] https://noqreport.com/2021/05/21/dr-christiane-northrup-explains-risks-of-covid-vaccine-spike-protein-shedding/

[460] Id.

[461] https://www.fda.gov/media/89036/download (August 2015)

[462] https://www.algora.com/Algora_blog/2021/10/04/pfizer-confirms-covid-vaccinated-people-can-shed-spike-protein-and-can-harm-the-unvaccinated (Oct. 24, 2021)

[463] Dr. Philippe VanWelbergen interviewed by Dr. Jane Ruby, https://drjaneruby.com/live-shedding-confirmed-the-jabbed-are-vaccinating-the-unjabbed/ (July 2022)

[464] https://stevekirsch.substack.com/p/are-100-dead-us-airline-pilots-trying (Dec. 12, 2021)

[465] Jack Bingham, https://www.lifesitenews.com/news/delta-airlines-pilot-dies-mid-flight-days-after-vaccination-report/ (Oct. 14, 2021)

[466] Daniel Villareal, https://www.newsweek.com/delta-denies-rumor-pilot-who-died-covid-vaccine-mid-flight-1638335 (Oct 12, 2021)

[467] Brian Shilhavy, https://healthimpactnews.com/2022/millions-of-american-lives-in-danger-as-airline-pilots-suffer-heart-problems-from-mandatory-covid-vaccines/ (April 26, 2022)

[468] Michael Nevradakis, https://childrenshealthdefense.org/defender/pilots-injured-covid-vaccines-speak/ (May 6, 2022)

[469] J.D. Heves, https://www.naturalnews.com/2022-04-29-squawk-7700-emergency-alerts-up-12400-percent-covid-vax-5g.html (April 29, 2022)

[470] Michael Nevradakis, https://childrenshealthdefense.org/defender/pilots-injured-covid-vaccines-speak/ (May 6, 2022)

[471] https://community.covidvaccineinjuries.com/cody-flint-33-year-old-pilot-severe-adverse-reaction-to-pfizer-covid-vaccine/ (March 9, 2022)

Chapter 32
Why Many Have Not Heard This Information Before: Reason #2

"The rights of every man are diminished when the rights of one man are threatened."
The late President John F. Kennedy

One question raised by many health care professionals addressed in Part 1 was: *"Why have we not been told this information before?"* It was suggested that there were three main reasons, the first of which was addressed in Part 1: *massive censorship, propaganda and suppression of data and other critical information* by the entire medical industrial complex. That includes government and international agencies and officials, major media (including the social media giants), vaccine manufacturers, governing medical boards, major medical publications and others who stand to benefit from promoting the COVID shots as safe and effective, such as health care institutions and investors like Bill Gates. Gates wields enormous influence over the World Health Organization, since his foundation is WHO's second largest donor.[472] He is on record as acknowledging that vaccines have been a highly profitable investment, yielding about a 20 to 1 return on his money.[473] Now that you have been made aware in this book of many kinds of evidence that have been censored from major media platforms, "fact-checked" and labelled as "misinformation," you can better understand the second reason why you have not been told much of this information before.

Reason #2: *The WHY behind the censorship, propaganda and suppression of information is massive* **CORRUPTION.** *The medical industrial complex had to try to hide their fraud, collusion, other crimes, as well as their real agenda, by labelling as "misinformation, disinformation or conspiracy theory" anything that caused "vaccine hesitancy" or*

WHY MANY HAVE NOT HEARD BEFORE: REASON #2

contradicted their official narrative. They had to de-platform alleged "misinformation spreaders" from social media to minimize the reach of their messages. They deployed an army of pro-vaccine biased "fact-checkers" to attack, demean and claim that the alleged misinformation spreaders' information was false and had been de-bunked.

The way they have gone about seeking to silence all voices that contradict the messaging they want people to hear reveals collusion and corruption in the activity of the Trusted News Initiative (TNI), discussed briefly in Part 1. The TNI is a perfect example of collusion of many of the above players to keep the medical community and the general public from knowing the truth about the COVID vaccines as well as "all things COVID." Among those involved in TNI are *The New York Times, The Washington Post,* the Associated Press (AP), Reuters, Google, Youtube, Twitter, CBC/Radio Canada, Microsoft, the BBC and many more networks, stations and print media.[474]

They are not even trying to hide their collusion to violate people's rights of freedom of speech by controlling the flow of any information that is contrary to their official narrative. Their website states that they are a "global partnership bringing together organisations across media and technology to tackle harmful disinformation in real time."[475] It also states: "Partners alert each other to high-risk disinformation so that content can be reviewed promptly by platforms, whilst publishers ensure they don't unwittingly share dangerous falsehoods." Such partnership and collaboration may sound like laudable efforts, but when their objective is to control speech according to their own definitions of truth, fake news, misinformation or disinformation, and to violate the Constitutional rights of others by silencing all dissenting views, that becomes problematic. Attorneys love it when a defendant's own documents and statements make their case for an injured plaintiff!

The major media and social media giants have played an indispensable role in promoting the official narrative (i.e., propaganda) and censoring and de-platforming all dissenting voices, especially the brave doctors and scientists who have refused to go along with their lies. At the same time, the manufacturers, investors like Gates, and various others such as the regulatory agencies who also have a financial interest in the vaccines, are making a small fortune. All of the players in the medical industrial complex have their own reasons for "partnering" with other players "within the club." Money is not the only incentive.

The amount of solid information about the dangers of these shots that is available in the independent media is quite overwhelming. Many of the doctors, scientists and others who have been sounding the alarm have done countless interviews. Increasing numbers of whistleblowers are coming forth to expose what is really going on – from the pharmaceutical companies, the government, the military and the health care community. More and more people are being awakened every day to the truth and reality of what is going on, despite the attempts of the medical industrial complex to prevent them from finding out.

The first three parts of this book have presented a great deal of evidence not just of the harm caused by the shots, but also many lies, misrepresentations, manipulation of data, irregularities in the manufacturing and regulatory processes, conflicts of interest, and suppression of important information that would support claims of fraud and collusion, as well as racketeering, crimes against humanity, genocide, and various other violations of the law, including treason. There are mountains of other evidence. To cite every example of fraud, corruption or collusion by players in the medical industrial complex would take volumes. Below is a small sampling of other instances related to the COVID vaccines.

It is important for the entire health care community to understand the ways and degree to which the key players that influence their industry are deliberately jeopardizing health care providers' own livelihoods and the treatment they provide to their patients. It is actions like those discussed in this book that cannot help but to have significant impacts on the entire health care system. The level of corruption has broken the system. It remains to be seen how it will be re-built or reformed.

In May 2022, an international coalition of 17,000 physicians and medical scientists called the Global COVID Summit issued a formal Declaration. It was a scathing condemnation of the corruption that has destroyed scientific integrity and has led to what their coalition and many others assert has risen to the level of ***crimes against humanity***.[476] Because of who and what their Declaration represents, it is important to quote certain portions of it directly:

"We, the physicians and medical scientists of the world, united through our loyalty to the Hippocratic Oath, recognize that the disastrous COVID-19 public health policies imposed on doctors and our patients are the culmination of a corrupt medical alliance of pharmaceutical, insurance, and healthcare institutions, along with the financial trusts which control them. They have infiltrated our medical system at every level, and are protected and supported by a parallel alliance of big tech, media, academics and government agencies who profited from this orchestrated catastrophe.

"This corrupt alliance has compromised the integrity of our most prestigious medical societies to which we belong, generating an illusion of scientific consensus by substituting truth with propaganda. This alliance continues to advance unscientific claims by censoring data, and intimidating and firing doctors and scientists for simply publishing actual clinical results or treating their patients with proven, life-saving medicine. These catastrophic decisions came at the expense of the innocent, who are forced to suffer health damage and death caused by intentionally withholding critical and time-sensitive treatments, or as a result of coerced genetic therapy injections, which are neither safe nor effective . . . .

"The mission of the Global COVID Summit is to end this orchestrated crisis, which has been illegitimately imposed on the world, and to formally declare that *the actions of this corrupt alliance constitute nothing less than <u>crimes against humanity</u>.*"

The Declaration also sets forth a list of 10 demands or calls to action, including the following: "the COVID-19 experimental genetic therapy injections must end;" doctors should not be prevented from providing life-saving treatment; "the state of national emergency which facilitates corrupt and extends the pandemic" should be immediately stopped; and violations of First Amendment protections and medical censorship must stop.

It also called for government, medical agencies and pharmaceutical companies to be held accountable, specifically declaring:

> "Pfizer, Moderna, BioNTech, Janssen, Astra Zeneca, and their enablers, withheld and willfully omitted safety and effectiveness information from patients and physicians, and should be immediately indicted for fraud."

The corruption and calls for legal action are also the subject of a powerful paper cited in Part 1 entitled "Patient Betrayal: The Corruption of Healthcare, Informed Consent and the Physician-Patient Relationship," published online in the *Gazette of Medical Sciences* in March 2022.[477] It was written by a group of 19 physicians, attorneys and other experts, of which one of this book's contributing authors, Dr. James A. Thorp, MD, was the lead author. One of the stated purposes of that paper was to:

> "bring to the attention of the populace, healthcare workers and healthcare administrators that illegal and unconstitutional gag orders have been placed on all healthcare workers in the US, and to alert everyone that no healthcare worker can be trusted since they are under a gag order which renders informed consent null and void. **It is our intent to put governing bodies of healthcare workers on notice that they will be held accountable and lay legal groundwork for possible Racketeer Influenced and Corrupt Organizations Act (RICO) violations, collusion, and fraud. These potential criminal acts, exposed in a court of law, can pierce legal immunity of Big Pharma and others, and pierce any perceived immunity given to hospitals and organizations via the CARES ACT.**" (emphasis added)

Dr. Robert Malone, one of the founders of the coalition that issued the above Declaration, echoed the above sentiment. When commenting in July 2022 about the FDA's continuing lie that there are no effective treatments for COVID-19, he said: "It illustrates how deeply corrupt this entire system is. How deeply captured it is by the pharmaceutical industry, and it's beyond just the FDA and the CDC."[478]

Former neurosurgeon Dr. Russell Blaylock, who has written about the censorship and corruption in medical journals, as reported in Part 1,[479] has also condemned the corruption in the following terms:

> "The COVID-19 pandemic is one of the most manipulated infectious disease events in history, characterized by official lies in an unending stream led by government bureaucracies, medical associations, medical boards, the media, and international agencies."[480]

Dr. Pierre Kory, another of the brave physicians accused of spreading misinformation, has said that the regulatory agencies and the manufacturers "mischaracterized and manipulated the data and ignored safety signals." If the FDA had done its job, he said, the COVID vaccines should have been stopped by the second week of January [2021] when the number of deaths and injuries being reported reached the levels when a product is recalled.[481]

Another issue highlighted by Kory involves the pharmaceutical industry's control over the research papers in the major medical journals that they use to support the official narrative. One side of that is that the drug companies find doctors who will publish papers with their desired outcomes. The other side is to suppress and censor any papers that contradict their narrative, regardless of the quality of the science behind them. Kory wrote an excellent and scathing multi-part article on this subject entitled "The Criminal Censorship of Ivermectin's Efficacy By The High-Impact Medical Journals." [482]

He cites a book by Dr. Marcia Angell, former chief editor-in-chief of the *New England Journal of Medicine,* entitled *The Truth About the Drug Companies: How They Deceive Us and What to Do About It.* Kory wrote that Angell had "resigned because of what she described as the rising and indefensible influence being exerted by Pharma on the prestigious journal and its powerful affiliate societies." He quotes from her book: "'It is simply no longer possible to believe much of the clinical research that is published or to rely on the judgment of trusted physicians or authoritative medical guidelines.'" According to Angell, while many believe that the high prices of drugs are due to high research and development costs, the truth is that the drug companies are now "'primarily a marketing machine to sell drugs of dubious benefit,'" and "'big Pharma uses its wealth and power to co-opt every institution that might stand in its way, including the US Congress, the FDA, academic medical centres and the medical profession itself.'"

Kory also cites Dr. Aseem Malhotra, the British cardiologist quoted earlier who used to promote the vaccines based on what doctors were being told about them. Malhotra said in an interview: "the real scandal is that doctors, institutions and medical journals collude with industry for financial gain and the regulators fail to prevent misconduct by industry." Malhotra also said: "We have a wealth of evidence of the fraud that's been committed by the pharmaceutical industry over the years, but for them it's the cost of business, because even though they've committed fraud… in almost all of those cases, nobody got fired…"[483]

Another issue of alleged collusion is revealed by Dr. Michael Yeadon's comments on the choice of the spike protein by all four manufacturers of COVID vaccines used in the U.S. (Pfizer, Moderna, J & J and AstraZeneca). Part 2 discussed why Yeadon believes the choice of the spike protein to base these shots on was a very poor one that "violated all of the accepted rules for creating a safe and effective product."[484] In addition, he suggests that for all four companies to make the same poor choice is evidence of collusion.[485] He challenged his colleagues and fellow scientists to consider the likelihood that all four companies would make the same inferior choice. He says that no vaccine development team he was on would ever have picked the spike protein for these shots. Furthermore, and if they had competing groups, it was simply not possible that all four of those in competition would have made the same mistake. Yeadon concluded: "Not possible. It's collusion and malfeasance. They did it on purpose, knowing it would hurt you." *If there was collusion among the manufacturers themselves regarding that issue, would not the regulatory agencies also be complicit since they were directly involved in authorizing these shots?*

Another example of collusion and other wrongdoing is reflected in a report by Steve Kirsch of the Vaccine Safety Research Foundation.[486] He and others had conversations with vaccine experts at a major university about the data showing the dangers of the COVID vaccines. The experts said they could not dispute the data presented by Kirsch and his team. However, they said that "further conversations would be 'unproductive,' because the decision was made above their level so no amount of scientific evidence showing harm could change [the university's] decision to mandate vaccination for their students." In other words, the truth and science do not matter. They have chosen to "go along" with the official narrative and compromise their integrity. Kirsch also reported that his many other attempts to "engage in public discourse with anyone at other leading medical institutions were rejected or ignored."

One other example of collusion is the complicity of financial institutions in seeking to destroy those who dare to contradict the official narrative.

WHY MANY HAVE NOT HEARD BEFORE: REASON #2

According to attorney Jeff Childers, who represents many doctors, and Dr. Deborah Viglione, [487] many of the doctors who have spoken out about the dangers of the COVID shots have had their financial accounts targeted. Some accounts and lines of credit have been frozen or otherwise made inaccessible. In some cases, loans have suddenly and unexpectedly been called due, even when the person was current in their payments. These and other kinds of "financial warfare" against the doctors have made it difficult for them to pay their expenses.

In looking at the issue of corruption and collusion, it may surprise many to learn that Pfizer has a history of criminal and civil liability for various unlawful practices. In November 2020, a law firm released an article entitled "Crimes of COVID Vaccine Maker Pfizer Documented." [488] The article noted that its list offers only a "brief glimpse of Pfizer's track record for safety and ethics. ..." Pfizer's wrongdoings include both civil and criminal charges such as racketeering fraud, misrepresentation, using children as human guinea pigs without parental consent, bribing doctors, and paying kickbacks. In 2009, it was hit with the biggest fine in U.S criminal history, $2.3 billion, when it agreed to plead guilty to a felony violation "for misbranding [a drug] with the intent to defraud or mislead."

Consider the point in Part 1 that the COVID shots are not "vaccines," but rather, they are "gene therapy products," according to the FDA's own definitions and the acknowledgement by Moderna and Pfizer's partner BioNTech. Then consider the three main benefits stated in Part 1 that the manufacturers enjoyed by calling them "vaccines" instead of "gene therapy injections": 1) they gained full protection from liability from any damages caused by these shots; 2) they avoided the much more rigorous regulatory requirements of gene therapy products; and 3) they were able to gain much greater public acceptance because people are familiar with vaccines, but very unfamiliar with gene therapy products.

Fraud is defined as a deception or intentional misrepresentation of a material fact for the purpose of inducing someone to part with something of value or to give up a legal right. *In light of the above, and with your "jury hat" on, would you consider the labeling of these genetic therapy injections as "vaccines" to be a significant misrepresentation or fraud? What about the many other examples of data manipulation, use of misleading definitions, and mischaracterizations of their own data? If you* had known the real nature of these shots and the reasons for calling them "vaccines," would you have gotten the shots yourself or have recommended or administered them to others? To the extent there was fraud, misrepresentation or other deceptions that led to people receiving these shots, how can it be said that anyone who received them had given truly *informed consent*? The Nuremberg Code of 1947 was intended to ensure that people would never again be subjected to medical experiments without sufficiently informed consent, without any form of deceit, fraud, duress, or coercion.[489] It appears that the Code has been substantially violated by the COVID vaccination campaign.

In addition to what has already been said about the new "Future Framework" strategy in Part 2 and earlier in this Part 3, the entire process by which it came to be implemented is rife with irregularities and smacks of corruption. The FDA granted Emergency Use Authorization on August 31, 2022 for the new Pfizer and Moderna reformulated bivalent COVID shots. The next day the CDC's advisory committee and the CDC director gave their approval, and the rollout started very shortly thereafter.[490] Aside from the lack of any clinical trials, *where was the emergency? Was it perhaps only on the part of the manufacturers to keep their vaccine profits rolling in on a regular basis?*

Dr. Meryl Nass, MD, explained that this "fastest rollout of a new vaccine in world history … occurred in the only way it could possibly occur: by bending the rules, creating a new regulatory playbook and failing to obtain any human data for the new vaccines."[491] Nass noted that the FDA did not meet with its advisory committee before issuing its EUA, adding that "it is not hard to guess why." She also noted that members of its advisory committee "have been complaining about being given less and less information as they are being asked to sign off on vaccine programs for younger and younger ages." According to Nass, just weeks earlier, one of the committee members stated that "'the fix was in,' implying that the committee's deliberations were a sham." With no human trials, and only very limited and not very meaningful data on 8 mice, Nass quotes Dr. Peter Marks, the director of the FDA's vaccine center as saying: "'**The public can be assured that a great deal of care has been taken by the FDA to ensure that these bivalent COVID-19 vaccines meet our rigorous safety, effectiveness and manufacturing quality standards for** emergency use authorization.'" *What "rigorous safety, effectiveness and manufacturing quality standards" was he referring to, and where are the data and other documentation to support this statement?* For more information about this topic, see Nass's article.

Another concern related to possible corruption arises from the government's creation of the COVID-19 Community Corps, a "nationwide, grassroots network of local voices people know and trust to encourage Americans to get vaccinated" that was launched on April 1, 2021. They had initially recruited 275 founding members representing health professionals, community organizations, faith leaders, businesses, civil rights organizations, sports leagues, athletes and others to encourage their friends, family members and neighbors to get the COVID shots.[492] The government also allocated almost $10 billion for this effort.

This program raises several questions. *Why mount such a campaign to protect against what for most people was no more serious than seasonal flu?*[493] *Why is the government willing to spend almost $10,000,000,000 to get people vaccinated but has offered little or no compensation to help the countless hundreds of thousands or even millions who have been injured, and families whose primary breadwinner either died or is no longer able to work after getting the COVID vaccination? Why should the government spend almost $10,000,000,000 in taxpayer money to promote a product made by private for-profit companies that the government would then pay billions of dollars more to for their product, to distribute for "free" to the public?*

Ten billion dollars seems like quite an excessive amount of money for this kind of program. A Freedom of Information Act request might produce some interesting information about who received how much of that $10,000,000,000 and for what, and whether there were substantial payments to any person or organization that look "suspicious." *In other words, was this possibly a scheme to "buy" a lot of people's help in promoting a corrupt agenda?*

No discussion about the corruption of Big Pharma and the government agencies would be complete without including Robert F. Kennedy, Jr.'s book, *The Real Anthony Fauci: Bill Gates, Big Pharma and the Global War on Democracy and Public Health.*[494] That book thoroughly documents how Big Pharma has effectively captured the regulatory agencies that are the very entities tasked with the responsibility of overseeing their industry, and the deep levels of corruption they have engaged in over many decades. It also focuses on the corruption of Anthony Fauci and Bill Gates in particular, in their relentless promotion of vaccines that have had devastating impacts around the world. Conflicts of interest abound in this arena, but the parties have all been able to get away with their corrupt schemes because they faced no effective opposition – at least not until now.

It is impossible to do justice to the contents of Kennedy's book in one or two paragraphs. However, suffice it to say that even if a person reads only part of this lengthy exposé, their trust in Anthony Fauci, Bill Gates, Big Pharma and the regulatory agencies, especially when it comes to vaccines, will never be the same. Even Dr. Robert Malone, who has worked with these people for decades in vaccine development, said in his review of the book: "I thought I understood what was going on from an insider POV [point of view] ... But what this book clearly documents are the deeper forces and systemic, pervasive governmental corruption, that have led us to this point...."[495] The book led award-winning director, producer and screenwriter Oliver Stone to ask: "'Has American medicine truly become a 'racket,' as corrupt as a mafia organization?'"

Legal Actions

Fortunately, the tide is now turning, as the above Declaration and actions of the brave doctors speaking out against the official narrative reveal. *Will you be the next health care professional to join their ranks, if you have not already?* One step towards accountability was taken on July 12, 2022, when the Association of American Physicians and Surgeons Educational Foundation (AAPS) filed a lawsuit in federal court in Texas naming as defendants the American Board of Internal Medicine (ABOM), the American Board of Obstetrics & Gynecology (ABOG), the American Board of Family Medicine (ABFM) and Secretary of the U.S. Department of Homeland Security, Alejandro Mayorkas. In essence, the Complaint alleged that the defendants engaged in the following actions:

> "unprecedented campaigns to censor speech that they falsely disparage as 'misinformation' or 'disinformation'. Defendants wrongly misuse their authority in a politically partisan manner to chill speech critical of positions taken by Dr. Anthony Fauci, lockdowns, mask mandates, Covid vaccines and even abortion.

WHY MANY HAVE NOT HEARD BEFORE: REASON #2

Defendants have acted in an apparently coordinated manner, using similar timing and terminology, to censor those who exercise their First Amendment rights on issues of public concern."[496]

Defendant Mayorkas was named in the suit based on his department's creation of the "Disinformation Governance Board ('DSG') in order to censor disfavored information based on its content." That Board was never authorized by Congress.[497] Fortunately, the Board was inactivated very shortly after it was created, after much public outrage, and was disbanded in late August 2022.[498]

Other legal actions have also already been filed. People are starting to fight back. Many lawsuits have been filed seeking injunctions against mandates and others for damages incurred by those who lost their jobs for refusing the shots. In what may be the first case in the nation to be concluded involving mandates, a settlement for $10.3 million was reached in July 2022 in a case filed against the NorthShore University HealthSystem in the Chicago area. It was filed by more than 500 current and former employees whose requests for exemption from the employer's mandate on religious grounds were denied.[499] The employees who had been fired were also offered the opportunity to return to work. The attorney for the plaintiffs said: "This settlement should be a wake-up call to every employer that did not accommodate or exempt employees who opposed the COVID shots for religious reasons."

That is probably the tip of the iceberg when it comes to actions against hospitals and other health care institutions (as well as other employers) who imposed mandates on their staff. Imagine what a wave of successful such actions all over the country would do to the entire system and the jobs of all health care professionals still within it.

Attorneys and their expert witnesses have been gathering mountains of evidence of massive fraud, deception, corruption, censorship and suppression to an extent they have never seen before, culminating in what they consider to be crimes against humanity. Until the latter part of 2022, attorney Reiner Fuellmich spearheaded a group he co-founded in mid-2020 called the Corona Investigative Committee.[500] Its purpose was to investigate the bases for governments' unprecedented restrictions in response to COVID-19 and the damage done by their actions. The committee interviewed hundreds of physicians, scientists, attorneys and other experts all over the world about "all things COVID-19." They convened a "Citizens Grand Jury" laying out all of the evidence they have collected.

With reference to findings based on certain evidence that Fuellmich believes shows deliberate intent to harm, he says that "these findings in particular will have immense legal repercussions, immense, because once you arrive at the conclusion that they are doing this deliberately, intentionally ... the floodgates are open, in the United States, for punitive damages." Punitive damages can amount to many times more than the actual damages, and that, Fuellmich believes, **"is enough to dismantle the entire industry."**[501] As much solid evidence as all of the physicians accused of spreading misinformation have to back up all of their "alleged misinformation," it appears that Fuellmich and his team of lawyers and other experts have even more. Their evidence goes far beyond just the vaccines, even back to the origins of the COVID crisis.

In the fall of 2022, Fuellmich founded a new organization called the International Crimes Investigative Committee (ICIC) which expands the scope of the earlier committee.[502] The crimes against humanity by the wealthy elite extend far beyond COVID. In this new ICIC, Fuellmich also intends to "show concepts for overcoming the corrupt, collapsing system."

On December 6, 2021, a group of UK citizens, including former Pfizer V.P. and scientist, Dr. Michael Yeadon, filed a criminal complaint with the International Criminal Court (ICC) against 16 defendants, including Dr. Anthony Fauci, the CEOs of three vaccine manufacturers, Bill Gates, Tedros Adhanhom Ghebreyesus (Director-General of the World Health Organization), and others.[503] Two of the allegations in that complaint were *crimes against humanity and genocide* based on the unprecedented numbers of serious injuries and deaths following COVID vaccinations.

The ICC is an international tribunal located in The Hague, Netherlands which is governed by international treaty called the Rome Statute, to which more than 120 countries are signatories, including the United States. It purports to be an independent court that investigates crimes of international concern, which prosecutes cases only when a State is unwilling or unable to do so. However, the ICC still depends on a nation's law enforcement because the ICC does not have a police force of its own. At the time of this publication, the status of that Complaint is not known,

WHY MANY HAVE NOT HEARD BEFORE: REASON #2

but it sets forth some of the evidence upon which the action was filed. The link to that document can be found in an article by Leo Hohmann entitled "Whistleblower activists file complaint with International Criminal Court alleging Big Pharma, Gates, Fauci, UK officials committed crimes against humanity," which also presents some of the Complaint's main points.[504]

After reading the first two of three reasons that answer the question of why many have not heard much of this information before, you may be wondering: *do these people not care about all the suffering and devastation they are causing, both individually and to the nation as a whole?* As difficult as it may be to believe, the answer to that is *no, they do not care*, at least not the ones at the higher levels.

The "why" behind that is explained in Part 4, the next and final part in this book. It focuses on the "big picture" that "all things COVID" fit into, and why there has been such an unrelenting push for everyone in the world to get vaccinated. It also addresses some of the most controversial issues, such as whether or not these shots can change DNA, and what is actually in the COVID shots, including reports of undisclosed substances.

---

[472] Julia Crawford, https://www.swissinfo.ch/eng/does-bill-gates-have-too-much-influence-in-the-who-/46570526 (May 10, 2021)

[473] Matthew J. Belvedere, https://www.cnbc.com/2019/01/23/bill-gates-turns-10-billion-into-200-billion-worth-of-economic-benefit.html (Jan. 23, 2019)

[474] https://www.trialsitenews.com/a/covid-19-censorship-trusted-news-initiative-to-decide-the-facts (June 25, 2021)

[475] https://www.bbc.com/beyondfakenews/trusted-news-initiative/about-us/

[476] https://globalcovidsummit.org/news/declaration-iv-restore-scientific-integrity

[477] Thorp JA, Renz T, Northrup, C, Lively C, Breggin P, Bartlett R, et al. Patient Betrayal: The Corruption of Healthcare, Informed Consent and the Physician-Patient Relationship. G Med Sci. 2022; 3(1): 046-069.https://www.doi.org/10.46766/thegms.medethics.22021403

[478] Dr. Robert Malone, Dr. Pierre Kory and Dr. Richard Urso interviewed by Del Bigtree, https://thehighwire.com/videos/malone-urso-kory-stop-vaccinating/ (July 15, 2022)

[479] Blaylock RL. COVID UPDATE: What is the truth?. Surg Neurol Int 22-Apr-2022;13:167. https://surgicalneurologyint.com/surgicalint-articles/covid-update-what-is-the-truth/

[480] Id.

[481] https://rumble.com/v1bp4ez-guilty-are-now-hiding-humanitarian-catastrophe-dr.-perrie-kory.html (July 9, 2022)

[482] https://pierrekory.substack.com/p/the-criminal-censorship-of-ivermectins (Sept. 16, 2022)

[483] https://twitter.com/DrAseemMalhotra/status/1542572960535429122 (June 30, 2022)

[484] https://media.mercola.com/ImageServer/Public/2022/August/PDF/bivalent-covid-vaccine-pdf.pdf (Aug. 22, 2022)

[485] Id.

[486] https://www.skirsch.com/covid/Refuse.pdf, p. 11

[487] Personal communication between Jeff Childers and Dr. Deborah Viglione (Sept. 2022)

[488] Matthews & Associates, https://www.dmlawfirm.com/crimes-of-covid-vaccine-maker-pfizer-well-documented/ (Nov. 18, 2020)

[489] https://encyclopedia.ushmm.org/content/en/article/the-nuremberg-code

[490] https://merylnass.substack.com/p/the-high-speed-bivalent-covid-boosters (Sept. 6, 2022)

[491] Id.

[492] https://www.hhs.gov/about/news/2021/04/01/hhs-launches-nationwide-network-trusted-voices-encourage-vaccination-next-phase-covid-19-public-education-campaign.html

[493] Peter R. Breggin, MD & Ginger Ross Breggin, *COVID-19 and the Global Predators: We are the Prey* (2021), p. xiv

[494] Robert F. Kennedy, Jr., *The Real Anthony Fauci: Bill Gates, Big Pharma and the Global War on Democracy and Public Health*, Skyhorse Publishing (2021)

[495] Ibid, in the endorsement section at the front of the book.

[496] https://aapsonline.org/judicial/aapsedfnd-v-abim-abog-abfm-dhs-7-12-2022.pdf, p. 1-2.

[497] Ibid., p. 4, 18

[498] https://www.dhs.gov/news/2022/08/24/following-hsac-recommendation-dhs-terminates-disinformation-governance-board

[499] https://www.theblaze.com/news/illinois-hospital-system-to-pay-10-3-million-in-settlement-with-workers-over-covid-19-vaccine-mandate (Aug. 1, 2022)

[500] https://corona-investigative-committee.com/

[501] Reiner Fuellmich: "New Findings…Enough to Dismantle the Entire (VAX) Industry." https://www.bitchute.com/video/M0vmjVc5mkQM/ (Jan. 1, 2022).

[502] Reiner Fuellmich interviewed by David Sorenson, https://www.stopworldcontrol.com/fuellmich-update (Oct. 1, 2022)

[503] Dr. Joseph Mercola, "Will These People Be Charged With Genocide?" https://takecontrol.substack.com/p/genocide?s=r (Jan. 23, 2022)

[504] https://leohohmann.com/2021/12/17/whistleblower-activists-file-complaint-with-international-criminal-court-alleging-big-pharma-gates-fauci-uk-officials-committed-crimes-against-humanity/ - more-8418

PART 4

THE "BIG PICTURE" THAT "ALL THINGS COVID" FIT INTO

including

WHAT IS IN THE VACCINES?

"The greatest tyrannies are always perpetrated in the name of the noblest causes."

Thomas Paine

English-American writer whose pamphlet "Common Sense" inspired the Declaration of Independence

ACCESS TO HYPERLINKS *of* ONLINE REFERENCES

For easy access to hyperlinks for all of the online references cited in this book, use the QR code on the left or the "Endnotes Hyperlinks" button at www.SallySaxon.com.

Chapter 33
Why Many Have Not Heard This Information Before:
Reason #3

"If you think we're fighting a virus, you're going to act like a victim. If you think we're fighting a war, you're going to act like a warrior." [505]

Dr. Lee Merritt, MD
Former Navy physician and surgeon / Orthopaedic & Spinal Surgeon
Past president of the Association of American Physicians and Surgeons

The first three parts of this book have discussed why the COVID shots are not vaccines, why they were never necessary in the first place, the great harm they have caused and how ineffective they have been. It also raised the issue of why so many health care professionals and scientists have been willing to risk everything to warn people of the dangers of these shots. It also discussed the first two of three reasons why many health care professionals have not heard this information before: ***massive censorship, propaganda and coverups of widespread and pervasive corruption and collusion within the entire medical industrial complex.***

This last part of this book pulls back the cover from the "big picture" that COVID fits into, and why there has been such an unrelenting push for everyone in the world to get vaccinated. It also addresses some of the most controversial issues about what is actually in the COVID shots, whether or not these shots can change DNA, reports of undisclosed substances in the vaccines, and whether there are other non-health purposes these shots may be serving. That brings us to the third reason why many have not been told this information before.

Reason #3 is the deeper "why" behind the censorship, propaganda and corruption: ***there is a much bigger agenda of those behind the push to inoculate the entire planet with the COVID and other vaccines.*** If you think that sounds like a "conspiracy theory," that should soon be dispelled.

Without understanding the big picture, it is impossible to really understand "all things COVID," and why the medical industrial complex has been so obsessed with what they called a "vaccine" as the sole strategy to end the COVID crisis. They refused to consider therapeutics, much less to embrace the early treatment protocols developed by several physicians that have been proven to work for literally untold hundreds of millions of people all over the world. Instead, they claimed there was no treatment for COVID, and even labelled some of the World Health Organization's "essential medicines" as dangerous and ineffective. They have ignored all of the warning signals that have been blaring from their own early warning system, VAERS, since the early weeks following the rollout. The physicians who have dared to warn the public of these dangers even before the rollout have been demonized, vilified and threatened with the loss of their license and board certifications. Several have already suffered such losses. Throughout this book, this question has been continually asked: **WHY?**

This is where the issue of *motive* arises because the government's strategies regarding all things COVID make no sense. *Why would a government, the major media (including social media giants), the governing medical boards, the major medical publications, and health care institutions resort to draconian and totalitarian tactics like censorship, demonizing, threatening and punishing dedicated physicians who were actually saving countless of lives and avoiding hospitalization and death of their patients?* Anthony Fauci and the others all have claimed to be following the science, yet they have turned science on its head. It seems that everything has been turned upside down when it comes to health care. **WHY?**

THE BACKGROUND OF PART 4

The answer to the "why" questions presented throughout this book requires a little background that will provide some important perspective on these issues. Since the mid-1990's, off and on, and after retiring from law practice not long after that, I have literally spent thousands of hours researching what is really going on in the world. I wanted to understand why things were the way they were, because certain things did not make sense to me. Since lawyers are trained to think logically (or at least they used to be), when logic is absent, I want to know why. ***What is the motive behind something that does not make sense?***

What I found was not what I expected. I truly wanted it not to be true, just like I felt about what I was finding out about the COVID "pandemic" and the shots. It created a major cognitive dissonance for me. As explained earlier, cognitive dissonance has been defined as "the mental discomfort that results from holding two conflicting beliefs, values, or attitudes."[506] For me, it was more than merely "mental discomfort" – it was a powerful motivation to pursue the issue until the confusion was resolved.

Perhaps many readers of this book have been experiencing a similar disconnect between what you have read in this book and what you had previously been told or believed about COVID and the vaccines. I can empathize. My experience was that staying in denial or in that place of confusion was the easier path – but only for awhile. The price of staying in that uncomfortable state became increasingly higher. I really did want to know the truth, wherever that would lead, so I pressed on. The more I researched, the more difficult it was to accept what I found. Some things seemed too difficult to believe. At some point, the amount and credibility of the evidence was just too compelling to deny. The same was true with the evidence about the COVID vaccines.

My research of the past few decades has taught me that what is really going on in the world is like a huge jigsaw puzzle with millions of pieces and a big picture. I also discovered it is impossible to understand what is really going on without seeing that big picture. Once you see it, pieces of the puzzle start to fall into place. You start connecting many seemingly unconnected pieces – representing situations, events and people.

Then you discover that many things are not at all as they appear to be, and that many things you have believed to be true actually are not.

COVID-19 is only one piece (or section) of that puzzle, but it is a big and very important one. Trying to understand COVID (or anything else that is going on) without seeing the big picture it fits into is like trying to put together that huge jigsaw puzzle without knowing what the picture is. *More dangerous yet* is not even trying to figure out what it is, or not even realizing that there ***is*** a big puzzle with a big picture that reveals what is really going on.

As stated in Part 1, we should all be able to believe what our government, the major media and the drug manufacturers tell us about issues as important as our health, especially in matters of life and death. But sadly, we cannot. All of the evidence presented in the first three parts of this book, taken together, reveals that we have all been lied to and deceived about "all things COVID" from the very beginning. We have been massively betrayed by those we trusted to look out for our best interests.

Health care professionals have been unconscionably forced into a position between the proverbial rock and a hard place. They have been forced to make choices between submitting to the will of the "powers that be" and violating their Hippocratic oath in order to keep their jobs, or standing up to a corrupt system and risk losing their jobs, their reputations and their credentials. Perhaps some never even questioned whether what they were directed to do was right or wrong.

The devastation resulting from "all things COVID" is not simply a result of bad judgment or policies, honest mistakes, incompetence or even greed. That is what at least many of the doctors, scientists and other experts accused of "spreading misinformation" discovered long ago. *What motivated them to risk everything?* It was not just their professional and ethical responsibilities to give their patients the best care they possibly could, based on what they knew to be effective. It was also what they knew or came to find out about the underlying motives and agenda of the people at the higher levels of the pyramid who have been promoting the false "safe and effective" narrative.

That same motivation is what is at the heart of this book. Two physicians teaming up with a retired attorney who saw a desperate need for the other side of the story to be heard by the health care community so that they, too, can find healing, restoration, and freedom from the effects of the trauma that COVID has inflicted upon them. They can even have a fresh start in life.

If everyone had known even some of the information presented in this book, or similar information freely and easily available from many other sources, it is highly doubtful that many people would have chosen to get these shots – even if mandated by their employer. *Is any job really worth it if one of the conditions of keeping it is getting a shot that may result in a person not even being able to continue performing that job, or worse?* If you have not already formed an opinion on that point, hopefully you will by the end of this Part 4.

WHY MANY HAVE NOT HEARD BEFORE: REASON #3

WHAT IS THE "BIG PICTURE" THAT COVID-19 FITS INTO?

The thousands of hours I have spent researching the big picture have been focused on various aspects of this ***foundational question: is there really a sinister agenda for world control planned by the wealthiest elites of the world? Do they really own or control the largest corporations (including Big Pharma), governments, the major media and practically every sector of society? Or is that just a conspiracy "theory," as the major media love to use as a means of deflecting various truthful reports? If there is such an agenda, what is it and how do these globalist elites operate?***

If you believe this "conspiracy stuff" is just a "theory," how do you explain the following statement by David Rockefeller, one of the top people among the wealthy elites? In his book, *Memoirs*, he states:

> "Some even believe we are part of a secret cabal working against the best interests of the United States, characterizing my family and me as 'internationalists' and of conspiring with others around the world to build a more integrated global political and economic structure – one world, if you will. If that's the charge, I stand guilty, and I am proud of it." [507]

The globalists used to be very secretive about their plans and kept them hidden from the general public. But in recent years they have brought their plans out much more into the open. Some think it is because the elites have come so close to finally achieving their big goal of global government, and believe that people of the world are now more open to it. Whatever their reason, they have spent decades employing various ways of conditioning people's minds to be ready to accept their plans, **without the masses even realizing how their minds were being influenced by various psychological methods.** The globalists have various strategies and tactics for accomplishing their global government and authoritarian control. However, their plans go far beyond just authoritarian-type control, as will be discussed below.

You may be aware that in January, 2022, the Biden administration proposed several amendments to the regulations of the World Health Organization (WHO) that would have, in essence, handed over our national sovereignty to that international body. Those amendments were to be voted on during the WHO Assembly held May 22-28, 2022. Apparently, all but one were withdrawn prior to a vote due to massive worldwide opposition.[508] But the fact that any American governmental administration would even propose such amendments should tell you all you need to know about the loyalties of that administration and those controlling it behind the scenes.

One of the worst of the proposals *would have removed the right of a country to object* to a declaration of health emergency by the WHO Director-General. That would encompass all of the enforcement measures that would follow, including involvement by various international agencies. That would, in essence, nullify our Constitutional and other legal rights, and bring in international agencies to enforce the declaration. The potential abuse of that authority by one person as a weapon or means of coercion against a country for political or other sinister purposes is undeniable. As if that were not concerning enough, that position is currently held (in fall of 2022) by someone whose loyalties and ideologies are not exactly favorable to the United States.[509]

Despite the withdrawal of those amendments to the WHO regulations, this battle is not over yet. These people still want a global Pandemic Treaty. Two very good resources for more information about this attempted power grab are James Roguski (www.LeaveTheWHO.com) and Dr. Peter Breggin, MD (www.Breggin.com).

The importance of the above foundational question for you is that it goes to the issue of your ability to believe two key points: 1) that those pushing the vaccines could possibly be deliberately acting against the best interests of the masses of people they purport to serve and protect, and 2) that these elites will lie, deceive, kill and do whatever is necessary to achieve their objectives.

This foundational question goes to the **motives of those at the top who have been directing "all things COVID," including the vaccine campaign.** Their real motives are very difficult to accept without knowing the big picture and seeing where COVID fits into it. As difficult as it is for many to believe, **there is *overwhelming evidence* that COVID was an "engineered crisis."** It was all planned. Countless experts agree. If you are not already aware of the compelling evidence of that, you are encouraged to read some of the reports at www.StopWorldControl.com/proof. Other resources to help you understand how it was planned and coordinated include the book by Dr. Peter Breggin and Ginger Ross Breggin entitled *COVID-19 and the Global Predators: We are*

WHY MANY HAVE NOT HEARD BEFORE: REASON #3

the Prey, published in 2021, or the book *COVID Operation: What Happened, Why It Happened and What's Next* by Pamela Popper and Shane Prier.

Also, in mid-2023, I plan to release the Updated and Expanded Edition of my own book, *Globalists on Trial: The Hidden Agenda to Destroy America From Within*.[510] It deals with the big picture and discusses several other key puzzle pieces besides COVID, such as the climate change narrative, and how the globalist elites operate. For example, it discusses how and why the elites engineer crises like a pandemic, or the *perception* of one, to advance their agenda.

The issue of pre-planning raises more issues: ***WHY would they do this? How could anyone be so cruel? And how could they actually pull off a fraud of such magnitude that upended the lives of billions of people all over the world?*** It all goes back to the big picture.

That issue is outside the scope of this book, but it is important to address it very briefly. It provides a very different lens through which to see the issues of vaccine safety, and why the government has refused to approve the proven treatments that countless doctors have been using with great success for well over two years.

Anyone who looks objectively at even just some of the evidence in this book cannot help but realize that *something is very wrong with the official COVID narrative*. Unfortunately, it goes beyond poor judgment, greed, incompetence, and even the desire to control the world.

One example of what was wrong was reflected in the October 2020 email quoted in Part 1 from former NIH director Francis Collins to Anthony Fauci. Collins spoke of the need for a "a quick and devastating published takedown" of the premises of the Great Barrington Declaration that had been signed by one Nobel Prize winner and three medical professors from Harvard, Stanford and Oxford whom Collins labelled as "fringe epidemiologists." That Declaration was also signed by tens of thousands of doctors, public health scientists and others expressing concerns and offering a better approach to the COVID crisis. The "devastating takedown" was necessary, Collins said, because the Declaration had been "gaining traction."

This is the same disdain and contempt with which Fauci, the CDC, the major media and others have treated the many physicians, scientists and other experts they have accused of "spreading misinformation."

Hopefully by now, if you have read the first three parts of this book, you have come to the conclusion that the real "spreaders of misinformation" are the elites and their supporters who have been promoting the "safe and effective" narrative. These elites think they know what is best for the rest of us. They do not think like "normal" people, as will be shown below. They have been lying and hiding their real agenda and many things they do not want the public and the health care community to know.

---

[505] Dr. Lee Merritt, https://tehamafreedom.org/2021/09/26/ltc-theresa-long-m-d-affadavit-military-injunction-to-stop-the-shot-mandate/comment-page-1/ (Sept. 26, 2021)

[506] Kendra Cherry, https://www.verywellmind.com/what-is-cognitive-dissonance-2795012 (July 29, 2022)

[507] David Rockefeller, *Memoirs*, p. 405

[508] https://www.lifesitenews.com/news/world-health-organization-temporarily-withdraws-controversial-us-amendments-to-proposed-treaty/ (May 26, 2022)

[509] Peter R. Breggin MD and Ginger Ross Breggin, https://breggin.com/article-detail/post_detail/Tedros-Introduces-Globalist-Plan-to-Take-Over-World-Health-Systems (May 6, 2022)

[510] The *Updated & Expanded Edition* of *Globalists on Trial* will be available on Amazon.com when released in mid-2023.

For more info about the Updated & Expanded Edition of

GLOBALISTS ON TRIAL
The Hidden Agenda to Destroy America From Within

Expected to be available in mid-2023.
To receive notification when it becomes available, sign up at:

www.GlobalistsOnTrial.com

Chapter 34
The "Great Reset" & The Globalists' New World Order

The connection between COVID-19 and what the wealthy elites have been planning for the world is explained in part in a book entitled ***COVID-19: The Great Reset***. It was published in July 2020 and written by one of the top figures in this elite group, Klaus Schwab. He is the founder and Executive Chairman of the World Economic Forum (WEF), a consortium of the world's wealthiest and most powerful people and companies. The connection between COVID and a much bigger plan is evident in the very title of Schwab's book. In other words, the COVID-19 "pandemic" was a major stepping stone to their "Great Reset." It was an "opportunity" (which they created) to advance their long-planned "New World Order" – one of those many alleged "conspiracy theories" which is actually a "conspiracy *in fact*," as Rockefeller admitted.

Their vision of a New World Order is the globalist elites' dream. But for the rest of us it is a nightmare. That subject is also outside the scope of this book. But because COVID is a key part of their radical plans, it is important to know certain things about it to understand the role the "vaccines" play.

Since 1992, Klaus Schwab and the WEF have been training up "Young Global Leaders" (originally "Global Leaders of Tomorrow") in the wealthy elites' philosophy, vision and agenda of global governance and their plans for humanity. Some of the graduates of these programs include Bill Gates, Pete Buttigieg (American Secretary of Transportation and former Democratic presidential candidate), Justin Trudeau (Canadian Prime Minister), and Volodymyr Zelensky (President of Ukraine), just to name a few. Many of the "globalists" leading the "Great Reset" and "New World Order" are alumni of these two organizations. Whether or not all of the graduates of this training are committed to and involved in the radical agenda of the WEF remains to be seen. Some may not be.

Their plans include (but go beyond) a global government that eliminates national sovereignty and exercises total control over the masses. The authoritarian control we have experienced during COVID is only a small taste of what they have planned. According to a former WHO employee, the WHO apparently has had plans to use pandemics as a way to obtain their long-sought global control.[511] Remember the new powers that certain nations sought to give to the Director-General of the WHO to unilaterally declare an "emergency" in any nation, and impose whatever restrictions or measures he deems appropriate.

COVID and the New World Order. Many political leaders have commented on the opportunities that a crisis creates for a "New World Order." In a March 2022 speech to the Business Roundtable, Joe Biden said: "And now is a time when things are shifting ... there's going to be a *new world order*...."[512] In 1990, President George H.W. Bush said:[513] "We stand today at a unique and extraordinary moment. The crisis in the Persian Gulf...offers a rare opportunity ... Out of these troubled times, our fifth objective — a *new world order* — can emerge."

Australian officials have openly confirmed the COVID connection. For example, in 2020, a *Sydney Morning Herald* headline read: "Australia's COVID-19 inquiry presents a roadmap for a *new world order.*"[514] In July, 2021, a TV station in New South Wales said: "Today is the first full day of the *New World Order*," as it announced new restrictions: outdoor gatherings would be limited to 2 people; browsing in shops was not allowed; and only one person per household was allowed to do essential shopping.[515] New South Wales Health Minister Brad Hazzard said: "This is a world pandemic... a one in 100-year event. So you can expect ... transmission from time to time, and that's just the way it is. *We've got to accept that this is the New World Order.*"[516] *Do we?* How many restrictions on your personal liberties and your Constitutional and legal rights are *you* willing to *"just accept"*?

The Elites' New World Order Agenda and Underlying Worldview

The elites' agenda for humanity is ***unimaginable*** to most people. There are reasons to believe that the globalist elites will be stopped before they are able to *fully imple*ment their agenda, at least for a time, but that is a totally different discussion about the path the world is on that we have never been down before. However, unless and until that happens, it would be advisable to pay attention to what is being said by Klaus Schwab and other globalists involved in the World Economic Forum.

The elites' worldview, as well as what motivates them, causes them to think in a totally different way than the rest of humanity. They see the world and life itself through a totally different lens. By understanding their worldview and what motivates them, we can understand how and why they can ignore all the safety signals that should have brought a halt to the COVID vaccine campaign shortly after it started, or should never have started at all. We can also understand why they seem so heartless, not caring at all about the suffering that they could so easily have prevented or lessened. By understanding their worldview, we can also see why they would carry out such a relentless campaign of massive censorship, lies, deceptions, coverups, fraud, corruption and others crimes to advance their agenda.

Schwab and his colleagues in the WEF are now very open about many aspects of their agenda that used to be hidden, so this is not speculation or "conspiracy theory." Before he wrote *COVID-19: The Great Reset*, Schwab wrote *The Fourth Industrial Revolution*, published in 2016. That book's Foreword states: "the technologies driving the fourth industrial revolution will fundamentally transform the entire structure of the world economy, our communities and our human identities." Schwab then wrote:

> "It is in the biological domain where I see the greatest challenges … We are confronted with new questions around what it means to be human, …and what rights and responsibilities we have when it comes to changing the very genetic code of future generations." [517]

Probably the only people raising questions about what it means to be human are those who want to change it. ***Does any human being have any "rights" to change the genetic code of future generations?***-He has also said: "The difference with the Fourth Industrial Revolution is that it changes ***you -- if you take genetic editing***."[518] Schwab describes this revolution as the "fusion of technologies across the physical, digital, and biological worlds."[519] This shows that changing genetic codes through gene editing is an important component in the elites' plans. The mRNA technology is a potential delivery system and one of the means to bring about that fusion.

Schwab's close advisor, Yuval Noah Harari, is someone most of us have never heard of. However, he has significant influence with many heads of state and in shaping debates on issues even within governments. He considers himself a historian. His book *Sapiens,* about the history of mankind (through his lens), has sold millions of copies worldwide, and he is a popular speaker. His work has been praised by many high-profile people such as Barack Obama, Bill Gates, and Mark Zuckerberg. One of his comments about COVID is:

> "the thing they will remember from the COVID crisis is this is the moment when everything went digital. ... this was the moment when everything became monitored, *that we agreed to be surveilled all the time*...And maybe most importantly... this was the moment when *surveillance started going under the skin*, because really we haven't seen anything yet ... the *big process that's happening right now in the world is hacking human beings*."[520]

What? Did we agree to such surveillance? Being hacked? Surveillance under the skin? Harari explains that so far, we have had governments and corporations all keeping track of where we go, who we meet, movies we watch, etc., but "the next phase" is "surveillance under the skin." In fact, he said: *"having the ability to monitor people under the skin, this is the biggest game-changer of all."* He says "above all, governments want to know what's going on under our skin." **Why? What does he mean by that?**

To Harari, human beings are simply "biological algorithms" that can be "hacked." It does not matter if the algorithmic calculations that make everything work are done by a human or by artificial intelligence.[521] He believes that "99 percent of human qualities and abilities are simply redundant for the performance of most modern jobs."[522] No wonder he states that the "most important question in 21st-century economics may well be:

> "What should we do with all the superfluous people, once we have highly intelligent non-conscious algorithms that can do almost everything better than humans?"[523]

He asked: "How exactly will the future masters of the planet look like? This will be decided by the people who own the data. Those who control the data control the future...." He explains further:

> "control of data might enable human elites to do something even more radical than just build digital dictatorships. By hacking organisms, elites may gain the power to re-engineer

the future of life itself. Because once you can hack something, you can also usually also engineer it." [524]

Harari even goes beyond that and says that "free will is over," and that "we are really upgrading humans into gods, for instance, the power to re-engineer life."[525] In one speech entitled "Will the Future Be Human?" he said: *"We are probably one of the last generations of homosapiens...we will learn how to engineer bodies, and brains and minds. These will be the main products of the 21st century economy."* [526]

At a 2020 WEF conference, one session was called "When Humans Become Cyborgs." [527] The American Heritage dictionary defines a cyborg as "a person who is part machine, a robot who is part organic." In that "Cyborg" session, the moderator explained: "we want to talk about recent developments in brain-computer interface, and how that's really blurring the line between man and machine."

Do we want human beings trying to "play God?" *Is it a good idea to "fundamentally change" what it means to be a human and to let unelected, self-appointed wealthy elites change the genetic code for future generations?*

As revealed by Harari's statements, these wealthy elites and those who serve their agenda do not think the same way "normal" people think. ***Understanding this is a key to being able to believe that these people would actually hurt people and destroy entire countries in order to advance their agenda.*** Perhaps by now you have begun to see why countless people believe that the elites' radical new world order agenda is actually *evil,* including "all things COVID." "Normal" people cannot imagine anyone even wanting to do to others what these people have planned, or being so indifferent to terrible human suffering. That is why it is so difficult for many to believe our own high government officials and others in positions of power really do *not* have our best interests at heart – regardless of their words, why they would actually harm us – and then *not even care*, just as Dr. Robert Malone was quoted as saying in Part 1.[528]

They see a crisis as an opportunity to do things they could not otherwise get away with doing. Therefore, it behooves them to *create* various crises to help break through barriers that are hindering their agenda. They are able to do this and get away with it and not be held accountable because they have control over virtually every area of society, including all branches of government.

Until recently, very few people were willing to speak out and take a stand. But COVID has changed all of that, especially the vaccines. A motivated and growing army of health care professionals, scientists, and many others have dared to take a stand because our freedoms, our lives and our nation have never been at greater risk.

---

[511] "The Plan," a documentary, https://stopworldcontrol.com/proof/

[512] https://www.whitehouse.gov/briefing-room/speeches-remarks/2022/03/21/remarks-by-president-biden-before-business-roundtables-ceo-quarterly-meeting/ (March 21, 2022)

[513] https://www.washingtonpost.com/archive/politics/1990/09/12/bush-out-of-these-troubled-times-a-new-world-order/b93b5cf1-e389-4e6a-84b0-85f71bf4c946/ (Sept. 12, 1990)

[514] Anthony Galloway, https://www.smh.com.au/politics/federal/australia-s-covid-19-inquiry-presents-a-roadmap-for-a-new-world-order-20200522-p54vd3.html (May 23, 2020)

[515] https://coercioncode.com/2021/07/12/australia-tv-station-reports-today-is-the-first-full-day-of-the-new-world-order-as-it-reports-new-lockdowns-in-sydney/ (July 12, 2021)

[516] John Gideon Hartnett, https://bibliscienceforum.com/2021/07/12/nsw-health-minister-announces-start-of-new-world-order/ (July 12, 2021)

[517] Prof. Dr. Klaus Schwab, *The Fourth Industrial Revolution* (p. 23). Crown. Kindle Edition (2016)

[518] https://rumble.com/v131ynd-elon-musk-grimes-mother-of-musks-two-children-we-are-becoming-cyborgs.html (at the 27:52 mark)

[519] Schwab, *The Fourth Industrial Revolution*, (p. 1).

[520] Yuval Noah Harari, "The COVID Crisis was the Moment When Surveillance Went Under the Skin," https://rumble.com/vxyfo5-yuval-noah-harari-the-covid-crisis-was-the-moment-when-surveillance-started.html

[521] Yuval Noah Harari, https://ideas.ted.com/the-rise-of-the-useless-class/ (Feb. 24, 2017)

[522] Id.

[523] Id.

[524] Yuval Noah Harari, "The COVID Crisis was the Moment When Surveillance Went Under the Skin," (cited above)

[525] https://rumble.com/v11rfj4-the-great-reset-covid-19-beast-system-explained-a.i.-nano-tech-brain-chips-.html

[526] Yuval Noah Harari, "Will the Future be Human?" https://www.youtube.com/watch?v=hL9uk4hKyg4&t=0s

[527] https://rumble.com/vmh8gx-covid-injections-indeed-change-the-human-dna.html

[528] Dr. Robert Malone, Dr. Pierre Kory and Dr. Richard Urso interviewed by Del Bigtree, https://thehighwire.com/videos/malone-urso-kory-stop-vaccinating/ (July 15, 2022) (starting around the 16:35 mark)

Chapter 35
Advancing the Globalist Agenda by Deception

Mark Twain is often quoted as having said: "It is easier to fool someone than to convince them they have been fooled." His actual statement was: "How easy it is to make people believe a lie, and [how] hard it is to undo that work again." [529] Expressed either way, the point is the same. The truth of this has been borne out concerning "all things COVID."

If I had not done as much research as I have on these topics, I myself would probably find it difficult to believe that our own government, the major media and the entire medical industrial complex could possibly ever lie and deceive the entire country (and even the world) in so many ways about something as important as our health. Much less would they deliberately seek to harm us and destroy the country in the process ... *Or* **would** *they?*

What about those proposed amendments to the WHO regulations that would have relinquished our national sovereignty and brought us under the control of an unelected foreign national with enormous power over controls like mandates, lockdowns and consequences for those who do not comply? What about the Future Framework allowing new formulations of COVID shots without any clinical trials? What about the total rejection and censorship by the entire medical industrial complex of proven life-saving protocols? The first three parts of this book have raised many such questions that cast suspicion on the motives and the *modus operandi* of the people behind the COVID "vaccine" campaigns.

As is the case with all of their plans and schemes that I have studied over the years, the globalist elites must use deception to advance their agenda. **They know that if the people they seek to control knew what their real agenda was, few would ever support it or go along with it. Therefore, they have to use deceptive means.** They attach labels like "conspiracy theory" or "misinformation" to mislead people away from the truth. They love to make it look like a person telling the truth is the one who is lying. It is a classic strategy to deflect attention away from their own wrongdoing by accusing their opponent of the very thing they are doing.

Unfortunately, we are easily deceived, as the above Mark Twain quote suggests, unless we know the big picture, but even then people can still be deceived. In his book, *How Evil Works: Understanding and Overcoming the Destructive Forces That are Transforming America*, author David Kupelian says:

> "...there's one technique that reigns supreme as the king of all propaganda weapons -- lying. To make evil look good, and good appear to be evil, you have to lie. "The power of the lies is not so much in the little 'white lies" that are part of the fabric of most of our lives. **It's in the big lies. It's paradoxical, but we're more likely to believe big lies than small ones**."[530] (emphasis added)

He goes on to say that Adolf Hitler "taught that the bigger the lie, the more believable it was." Hitler was also known for saying that if you repeat a lie frequently, sooner or later, enough people will believe it.[531] This is precisely what the globalist elites have done during COVID. Actually, they have been telling big lies and repeating them over and over for many years on many issues. They are masters of lying, deception and mind control, and COVID brought them all to a new level. Since they control the major media, including the social media giants, it is easy to tell enough lies that create enough fear to lead people to comply with whatever they want people to do.

The big lies behind COVID have been too big for most people NOT to believe. The fact that life and death issues were involved made it even easier to pull off the deception, for reasons already explained. The more research I did about "all things COVID," the more evidence I found showing COVID to be an "engineered crisis," and that the "vaccines" were not what we were led to believe either.

On virtually every major point in the devastating COVID saga, the evidence reveals that the official narrative has been based upon one lie and deception after another. Just as Dr. Robert Malone was quoted earlier as saying:

> "They have been lying and lying and lying and lying. There are multiple layers of fraud going on...They're trying to get away

with the fact that there were multiple misrepresentations that this vaccine could get us to herd immunity… The lies keep coming. They don't stop. They don't care." [532]

The evidence continues to mount showing that a colossal fraud has been perpetrated against the whole world concerning "all things COVID." If only it were not true.

Unless and until the elite globalists are stopped, **those among them who are pushing these vaccines are counting on the majority of health care professionals to continue going along with their "emergencies" and "pandemics," recommending and administering their harmful injections and other protocols.** But patients – and everyone else – are counting on them to do the *right thing,* both for their health and in the fight against medical and political tyranny.

---

[529] Matt Seybold, https://marktwainstudies.com/easiertocon/ (June 10, 2022)

[530] David Kupelian, *How Evil Works: Understanding and Overcoming the Destructive Forces That are Transforming America* (Threshold Editions, a division of Simon & Schuster 2010), p. 14.

[531] Id..

[532] Dr. Robert Malone, Dr. Pierre Kory and Dr. Richard Urso interviewed by Del Bigtree, https://thehighwire.com/videos/malone-urso-kory-stop-vaccinating/ (July 15, 2022) (starting around the 16:35 mark)

Chapter 36
Can the COVID Vaccines Change a Person's DNA?

One of the most serious concerns about what is in the COVID-19 vaccines and how they work is whether or not they can change a person's DNA. If they can, obviously that has enormous and disturbing implications for humanity – both for people individually and society as a whole.

The medical industrial complex says that is impossible, and that claims to the contrary have been "de-bunked." However, if we "follow the science," the evidence shows there is definitely cause for concern. Remember the earlier evidence that the COVID shots are really ***gene therapy products, not vaccines.*** That is an important piece of the puzzle. ***Think about that for a moment: why would we need genetic material injected into our bodies to protect against a virus?***

Keep in mind that unreliable bias is likely to result in studies done by researchers funded directly or indirectly (such as through universities) by the pharmaceutical companies, government grants, major foundations or other non-profits that have a vested interest in the official narrative. That is true for researchers on any COVID-related topics.

There are at least two main issues to consider: 1) can mRNA and the vector vaccines (J &J) be intercalated into and alter a person's DNA?; and 2) if so, will it permanently change a person's DNA and be passed to future generations? According to Dr. Deborah Viglione, some are under the impression that the J & J was a safer alternative, but in reality, it directly enters the nucleus of the cell where the person's DNA resides.

One article on this topic is by Dr. Doug Corrigan, Ph.D., entitled "MIT & Harvard Study Suggests mRNA Vaccine Might Permanently Alter DNA After All," [533] dated March 16, 2021. Dr. Corrigan has a Ph.D. in Biochemistry and Molecular Biology, a master's in Engineering Physics (with a concentration in Solid State Physics), and a bachelor's in Engineering Physics.[534] He is also an innovator, has won many awards and has been named a "Super Solver" in the book *One Smart Crowd*. Like other experts whose research leads them to draw conclusions contrary to the official narrative, he has had his share of smears, but remember who the fact-checkers work for. In that article he explains:

> "...we've been told in no uncertain terms that it would be impossible for the mRNA in a vaccine to become integrated into our DNA, simply because 'RNA doesn't work that way.' Well, this current research which was released not too long after my original article demonstrates that yes, indeed, 'RNA does work that way'. In my original article, I spelled out this exact molecular pathway.
>
> "Specifically, a new study by MIT and Harvard scientists demonstrates that segments of the RNA from the coronavirus itself are most likely becoming a permanent fixture in human DNA... This was once thought near impossible, for the same reasons which are presented to assure us that an RNA vaccine could accomplish no such feat. Against the tides of current biological dogma, these researchers found that the genetic segments of this RNA virus are more than likely making their way into our genome. They also found that the exact pathway that I laid out in in my original article is more than likely the pathway being used...."

His original article referred to was dated November 2020, before the vaccine roll out, and before the EUA was granted. It is entitled "Will an RNA Vaccine Permanently Alter My DNA?" in which he described the reverse transcription (RT) process through which he believes this is possible.[535]

He explains why the RT process is even more likely to occur with *the RNA in the vaccine* than with the RNA in the virus itself which was used in the MIT-Harvard study. One of the possible outcomes of this, he explained, was how people receiving the mRNA injections "will almost inevitably develop autoimmune conditions which are irreversible, since this foreign protein antigen is now permanently hard-wired into the instructions contained in their DNA." This seems to be consistent with what doctors have reported as well after the vaccine rollout, as presented in Part 2.

The MIT-Harvard study Corrigan referred to in his March 2021 article was published in December 2020. It is entitled "SARS-CoV-2 RNA reverse-transcribed and integrated into human genome."[536] That study found "evidence that SARS-CoV-2 RNAs can be reverse transcribed in human cells by reverse transcriptase (RT) from LINE-1 elements or by HIV-1 RT, and that these DNA sequences can be integrated into the cell genome and subsequently be transcribed."

An update of that study was published in May, 2021 entitled "Reverse-transcribed SARS-CoV-2 RNA can integrate into the genome of cultured human cells and can be expressed in patient-derived tissues."[537]

> "…we found that DNA copies of SARS-CoV-2 sequences can be integrated into the genome of infected human cells. We found target site duplications flanking the viral sequences and consensus LINE1 endonuclease recognition sequences at the integration sites, consistent with a LINE1 retrotransposon-mediated, target-primed reverse transcription and retroposition mechanism. We also found, in some patient-derived tissues, evidence suggesting that a large fraction of the viral sequences is transcribed from integrated DNA copies of viral sequences, generating viral-host chimeric transcripts."

Another even later study, published in early 2022, is entitled "Intracellular Reverse Transcription of Pfizer BioNTech COVID-19 mRNA Vaccine BNT162b2 In Vitro in Human Liver Cell Line."[538] The abstract in that study states in part:

> "Our results indicate a fast up-take of BNT162b2 into human liver cell line Huh7, leading to changes in LINE-1 expression and distribution. We also show that BNT162b2 mRNA is reverse transcribed intracellularly into DNA in as fast as 6 h upon BNT162b2 exposure."

That study not only noted that the RT process was changing the RNA into DNA in only six hours, but also that a "possible mechanism for reverse transcription is through endogenous reverse transcriptase LINE-1, and the nucleus protein distribution of LINE-1 is elevated by BNT162b2."

Another paper that discusses the issue is entitled "mRNA vaccines: Why is the Biology of Retroposition Ignored?"[539] Regarding the claim that mRNA vaccines cannot alter DNA, the author says that the claim is widely stated in the literature, but it is "never supported by referencing any primary scientific papers that would specifically address this question." This was puzzling, he wrote, because of the work that had already been done on various aspects of retroposition that "clearly documents the frequent integration of mRNA molecules into genomes...."

---

[533] Dr. Doug Corrigan, https://www.algora.com/Algora_blog/2021/03/16/mit-harvard-study-suggests-mrna-vaccine-might-permanently-alter-dna-after-all (March 16, 2021)

[534] https://sciencewithdrdoug.com/about-me/

[535] https://sciencewithdrdoug.com/2020/11/27/will-an-rna-vaccine-permanently-alter-my-dna/ (Nov. 2020)

[536] Zhang L, Richards A, Khalil A, Wogram E, Ma H, Young RA, Jaenisch R. SARS-CoV-2 RNA reverse-transcribed and integrated into the human genome. bioRxiv [Preprint]. 2020 Dec 13:2020.12.12.422516. doi: 10.1101/2020.12.12.422516. PMID: 33330870; PMCID: PMC7743078, https://pubmed.ncbi.nlm.nih.gov/33330870/

[537] Zhang, L.; Richards, A.; Barrasa, M.I.; Hughes, S.H.; Young, R.A.; Jaenisch, R. Reverse-transcribed SARS-CoV-2 RNA can integrate into the genome of cultured human cells and can be expressed in patient-derived tissues. Proc. Natl. Acad. Sci. USA 2021, 118, e2105968118. https://pubmed.ncbi.nlm.nih.gov/33958444/ (May 25, 2021)

[538] Alden, Markus, et al, "Intracellular Reverse Transcription of Pfizer BioNTech COVID-19 mRNA Vaccine BNT162b2 In Vitro in Human Liver Cell Line," https://www.mdpi.com/1467-3045/44/3/73/htm?s=09 (Feb. 23, 2022)

[539] Domazet-Lošo T. mRNA Vaccines: Why Is the Biology of Retroposition Ignored? Genes (Basel). 2022 Apr 20;13(5):719. doi: 10.3390/genes13050719. PMID: 35627104; PMCID: PMC9141755. https://pubmed.ncbi.nlm.nih.gov/35627104

Chapter 37
Technologies Relating to DNA and Genetic Editing

There is much we still do not know about the COVID shots, both those that have already been administered as well as current and future ones for which there are no clinical trials or rigorous testing. Because of the lack of transparency already discovered on the part of the manufacturers, and what we know generally of the elites' plans, it is important to understand what technological capabilities exist and what technologies the manufacturers are using in other products that could potentially also be used in the COVID shots, if not already used. Technologies involving creation of "synthetic life forms,"[540] "recombinant DNA" (combining DNA from different sources) and "gene-editing" have been advancing for several years already. They have even made it possible to create *chimeras* – hybrid DNA from more than one species.

CRISPR/Cas9 is a genome editing technology that won its inventors a Nobel Prize in Chemistry. It enables users to make a simple "snip" in the genome which disables a gene and allows something else to be inserted in its place. They could even insert a DNA sequence the users have designed themselves according to certain genes they desire to have ("designer genes"). RNA can be used for transporting or reading the DNA "instructions."[541]

An article in November 2021 revealed that Moderna had entered into a partnership with Metagenomi, a CRISPR gene editing company.[542] The article reported:

> "...the partnership will involve in vivo treatment options for serious genetic diseases. Metagenomi will offer up access to its gene editing tools while Moderna will bring the expertise in mRNA and lipid nanoparticle delivery technologies."

It also said: "The companies plan to deliver their medicine where other gene editing companies have already established a precedent—the liver, using delivery tech Moderna already has. ..."

Pfizer has also been pursuing CRISPR gene-editing technology. Part of its website deals specifically with "Gene Therapy" and talks about gene editing, including the use of CRISPR and other technologies.[543]

It is important to make clear that these references in the Pfizer website and Moderna's partnership with Metagenomi *by themselves* are not proof of any definite connection between their COVID vaccines and gene editing. However, the point is that this technology is available to them, and it appears clear that they are either already using or intending to use this technology for other purposes. In light of other things we do know, it is wise to be cautious about things we do not know.

An earlier version of the Moderna website,[544] which can be found through the "Wayback Machine," explained its mRNA technology this way:

"Our Operating System
Recognizing the broad potential of mRNA science, we set out to create an mRNA technology platform that functions very much like an operating system on a computer. It is designed so that it can plug and play interchangeably with different programs."

Operating system? What kinds of "programs" can be "plugged and played?" Who decides? And who has control or access to this technology in a person's body? And more specifically, what "programs" has Moderna used in its COVID vaccines? Have its "program instructions" included anything more than to stimulate an immune response to SARS-CoV-2, as was represented to the public and the medical community? And for how long has the body been instructed to continue making the spike protein? There are many questions that most people in the health care community do not know the answers to about this technology and how the COVID vaccine manufacturers have used it in these shots.

The earlier website version describes its "mRNA medicines" as "the Software of life." In a 2017 TEDx talk entitled "Rewriting the Genetic Code," the Chief Medical Officer of Moderna, Dr. Tal Zaks, stated: "we are actually hacking the software of life."[545] The "software of life" is well-known to refer to DNA. He was presenting several good potential uses of this technology which the audience was excited to hear about.

It may well be that the potential use of such technology for good purposes is enormous. But the potential misuse for *evil ends* is equally enormous, raising serious moral and ethical concerns. It depends on who is in control of the technology, and the degree of freedom a person has to choose to use it or not – without being threatened with major adverse consequences, as with COVID vaccine mandates.

Considering the fact that the government and the manufacturers have been unusually keen on seemingly endless booster shots more than once a year, **does it make you wonder if there might be something more going on here than seeking to prevent or lessen the severity of a disease called COVID?**

The latter point also includes the issue of whether or not people are even aware or informed when the technology is being used. For example, there is a developing technology for "self-spreading" or "contagious" vaccines which do what their name reflects.[546] That is, such products can "vaccinate" people indirectly, similar to the shedding phenomenon discussed in Part 3. It may only take a very small percentage of the population to actually receive a "self-spreading" vaccination in order for the entire population to be effectively "vaccinated." The author of an article on that topic[547] concludes by saying: "Government-funded research of lab-engineered viruses to create contagious self-spreading vaccines that bypass the consent of citizens. *What could go wrong?*"

An extremely alarming Executive Order was signed by the Biden administration on September 12, 2022 entitled "Advancing Biotechnology and Biomanufacturing Innovation for a Sustainable Safe, and Secure American Bioeconomy."[548] One of the key features of this Order is:

> "We need to develop genetic engineering technologies and techniques to be able to write circuitry for cells and predictably program biology in the same way in which we write software and program computers; unlock the power of biological data, including through computing tools and artificial intelligence; and advance the science of scale-up production while reducing the obstacles for commercialization so that innovative technologies and products can reach markets faster."

In light of everything else we know, it appears that the Biden administration, or those controlling it, are trying to make this "transhumanist" agenda and its genetic engineering the "new normal." This Order also reveals that they intend to put significant resources into this effort. While the Order also has nice language about using such technology in an ethical and responsible manner, remember that they make their own definitions to suit their objectives. ***Do you trust them to use such technology ethically and responsibly?*** It may sound good on the surface, but the potential implications are far and wide, and not all are for good. ***Does this look like it might have Big Pharma's signature on it, to create new income streams paid for by the government?***

The subject of the available technology is one about which Karen Kingston, a biotech analyst who has served as a consultant in the pharmaceutical and medical device industry for many years, has much to say. She has expertise in analyzing clinical data, patents, federal regulations, and related matters, and has done extensive research into some of the nanotechnology issues surrounding the COVID vaccines. Kingston is also very familiar with the serious problems in the clinical trials and the contents of many relevant documents of the manufacturers and the regulatory agencies.

In October 2022 she began publishing a very eye-opening multi-part series on her substack platform entitled "Dismantling the Deceptions of the COVID-19 Story."[549] She has also been interviewed on various platforms about this subject matter.[550] Kingston's series covers in greater detail what she has found out about the mRNA virus, the spike protein, the technology introduced in the COVID vaccines and what it is does, gain-of-function research, hydrogels and other important related topics, including ones reported on below. These topics, and what Kingston reports on, involve some hard truths about what is going on in the bio-tech field, and how various issues are inter-related. These are issues that everyone needs to be aware of, but particularly the health care community, as they are increasingly impacting the entire field of health care.

---

[540]https://www.ted.com/talks/craig_venter_watch_me_unveil_synthetic_life/transcript?language=en (May 2010); see also Ian Sample, https://www.theguardian.com/science/2010/may/20/craig-venter-synthetic-life-form (May 20, 2010)

[541] http://www.crisprtx.com/gene-editing/crispr-cas9

542 Annalee Armstrong, https://www.fiercebiotech.com/biotech/moderna-finally-cracks-into-gene-editing-metagenomi-pact-thanks-irresistible-data (Nov. 2, 2021)

543 https://www.pfizer.com/science/innovation/gene-therapy/genes-as-medicines

544 https://web.archive.org/web/20220114040737/https://www.modernatx.com/mrna-technology/mrna-platform-enabling-drug-discovery-development

545 Dr. Tal Zaks, "Rewriting the Genetic Code," https://www.youtube.com/watch?v=AHB2bLILAvM

546 Aaron Kheriaty, https://brownstone.org/articles/contagious-vaccines-a-warning (June 16, 2022)

547 Id.

548 https://www.whitehouse.gov/briefing-room/presidential-actions/2022/09/12/executive-order-on-advancing-biotechnology-and-biomanufacturing-innovation-for-a-sustainable-safe-and-secure-american-bioeconomy/

549 https://karenkingston.substack.com/

550 For example, https://citizens.news/663687.html (Oct. 6, 2022)

Chapter 38
Contents of the Vaccine Vials: General Concerns & Blood Samples

There are several issues pertaining to the contents of the vaccine vials. Some involve certain listed ingredients, while others are *undisclosed* substances that reportedly have been found. Others involve ingredients for which the manufacturers claim "proprietary information" as their reason for non-disclosure. The problem with that in the pharmaceutical context is that it prevents a consumer from being able to give truly informed consent. It appears that we may know more about the contents of the vials from independent researchers than we do from the manufacturers. We authors cannot ourselves verify their results, but because multiple researchers worldwide have found the same or very similar things, we felt it was important to present this information.

General Concerns

There are several issues discussed earlier which raise concerns about the actual contents of the vials:

1) The concerns expressed by Dr. Michael Yeadon and former pharmaceutical company employees about the manufacturing process and the compliance issues.

2) The findings of the Paardekooper/Team Enigma research as to the significant inconsistencies in the safety profiles between different lots from the same manufacturer, and similar pre-rollout concerns expressed by the EMA regarding excessive and unacceptable variations in the % mRNA integrity. *Do such inconsistencies still exist in batches made after their research was done? What was causing the inconsistencies in the first place? Were there different ingredients or different doses, or did the inconsistencies result from something done at the place of administration?*

3) The way the clinical trials were conducted, and the way that EUA was granted based on manipulated trial data that was presented to the FDA.

4) The suspicion aroused by the government's bulldog determination to get everyone injected with these shots when a vaccine was not even necessary in the first place.

5) The fact that these shots are not actually vaccines, but "gene therapy" products, and the suspicions raised by such misrepresentation as to what might be in these injections.

6) Concerns arising from the FDA's new scheme after June 2022 eliminating clinical trials for any "reformulations" of COVID "vaccines."

7) What doctors doing autopsies and embalmers are finding in the bodies of deceased vaccinated persons that they have never seen before the COVID vaccine rollout.

Blood Samples Before and After COVID Vaccinations

One way of determining what is in the vials, and to determine if the vaccines are causing any abnormalities in the body, is through blood analysis using various kinds of microscopic or imaging equipment. Several doctors and researchers in many countries have examined blood samples of vaccinated patients, including samples both "before and after" vaccination from the same patient. Their findings are very similar and consistent. Dr. Barbel Ghitalla from Germany has been doing blood analyses for many years, and describes the rouleaux condition in her vaccinated patients as "severe." She has never seen anything like this before, and is afraid for her patients.[551]

Dr. Zandré Botha from South Africa has a Ph.D. in Alternative Medicine, Diploma in Integrative Medicine, and is a certified live and dry blood analyst. She has been examining patients' blood for over 15 years and uses advanced microscopic techniques. She says that more and more of her patients have post-COVID vaccine illnesses.[552] Figures 4 and 5 below are photos of one of her patient's blood samples before and after receiving a COVID shot. These were taken in 2021, so it was known at least that early what these shots were doing to people's blood. ***Dr. Botha also said that 100% of her cancer patients who got the shots and whose cancer had been in remission now have cancer again that is spreading.*** This is consistent with what pathologist Dr. Ryan

CONTENTS OF THE VACCINE VIALS: GENERAL CONCERNS

Cole has reported about cancers "taking off like wildfire" after COVID vaccinations because the lipid nanoparticles are shutting down certain pattern receptors.[553]

A study was published in August 2022 by three Italian surgeons who had done blood analyses on 1,006 patients who had developed various disorders after receiving the Pfizer or Moderna COVID shots, and an article in *The Epoch Times* in September 2022 reported on this study.[554] Figure 6 below shows a set of "before and after" vaccination photos from their study. Using dark-field microscopy, they found that 94% of those tested had abnormal blood samples:

> "Aggregation of erythrocytes were highlighted and exogenous point-like and self-luminescent particles in the dark-field were detected ... The alterations in the erythrocytes show a tendency to aggregation/disintegration, stacking in rouleaux, hemolysis, and other conditions suggestive for an important alteration of their zeta potential... With the hematological pictures we have presented here it is reasonable to expect reactivation of oncological disease along with blood circulation disorders."

The various kinds of foreign particles they observed had different shapes and sizes. Their study includes several photos showing the condition of the blood and the presence of foreign objects. They also observed that "The luminescence of those particles was markedly higher than that of oxygenated red blood cell walls." (See the section below on *Undisclosed Substances* concerning foreign objects found in the vaccine vials themselves.) In addition, they noted that the results of their study were very similar to those of Korean doctors who published their study in the same *Journal* in March 2022, essentially replicating the Koreans' results but with a much bigger sampling.[555]

A third set of "before and after" vaccination photos shown below in Figure 8 were taken by Dr. Felipe Reitz from Brazil.[556] Other photos of post-vaccination blood samples can be found in the same sources the photos in the figures below came from, as well as from various other sources, including *The Epoch Times*,[557] The German Working Group for COVID Vaccine Analysis,[558] a group of researchers from Korea,[559] and a group of Australian scientists. [560]

For the most part, the post-vaccination photos in the three different sets below primarily show the distinct rouleaux condition in the patients' blood. Less noticeable are various shapes and sizes of what the above and other sources have identified as "foreign objects." Other blood sample photos from some or all of these same sources show such objects more prominently, and the sources say these objects are not artifact or foreign material on the slide itself.

Figure 4. [561] Photo from Dr. Zandré Botha (South Africa) of a patient's blood BEFORE a COVID vaccination.

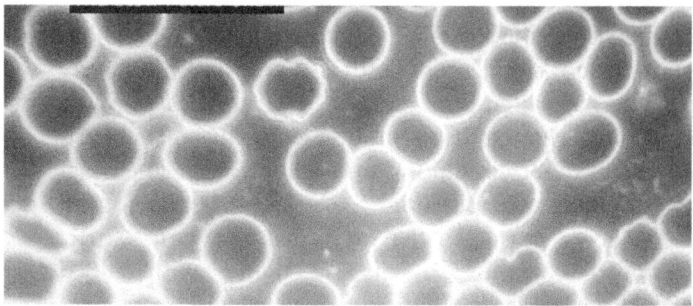

Figure 5. [562] Photo from Dr. Zandré Botha (South Africa) of the blood of the same patient as in Figure 4, AFTER a COVID vaccination

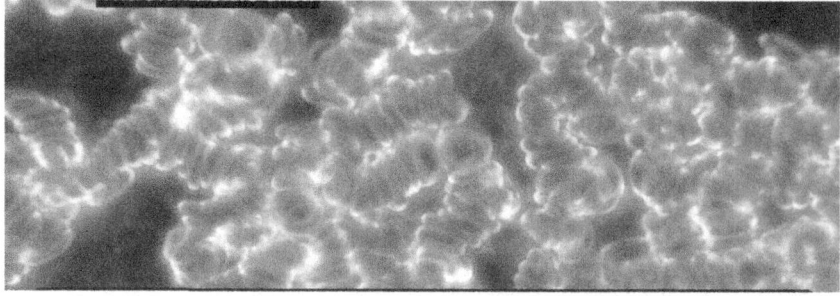

Figure 6. [563] Photos and original description below by Franco Giovannini, MD, Riccardo Benzi Cipelli, MD, DDS, and Gianpaolo Pisano, MD, OHNS (Italy). (These photos and the legend on the following page are displayed as "Figure 1" in their study referenced below.)

CONTENTS OF THE VACCINE VIALS: GENERAL CONCERNS

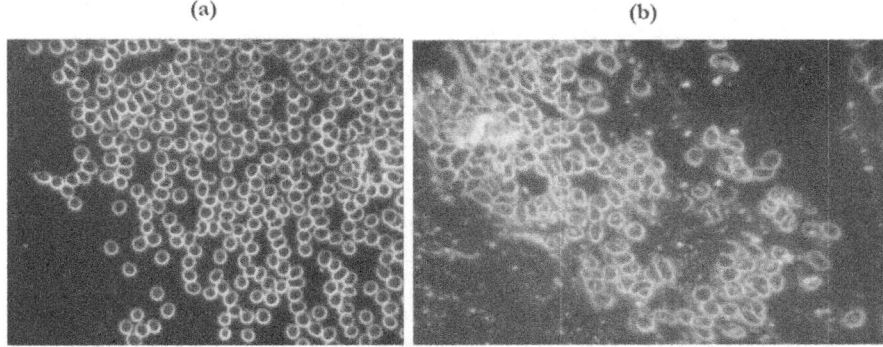

"These photos are at 40x magnification. At the left side, (a) shows the blood condition of the patient before the inoculation. The right side image, (b) shows the same person's blood one month after the first dose of Pfizer mRNA "vaccine." Particles can be seen among the red blood cells which are strongly conglobated around the exogenous particles; the agglomeration is believed to reflect a reduction in zeta potential adversely affecting the normal colloidal distribution of erythrocytes as see[n] at the left. The red blood cells at the right (b) are no longer spherical and are clumping as in coagulation and clotting. "

Figure 7. [564] Photos by Dr. Felipe Reitz (Brazil) using thermographic imaging, with his own descriptions (before VAX on the left, after VAX on the right.)

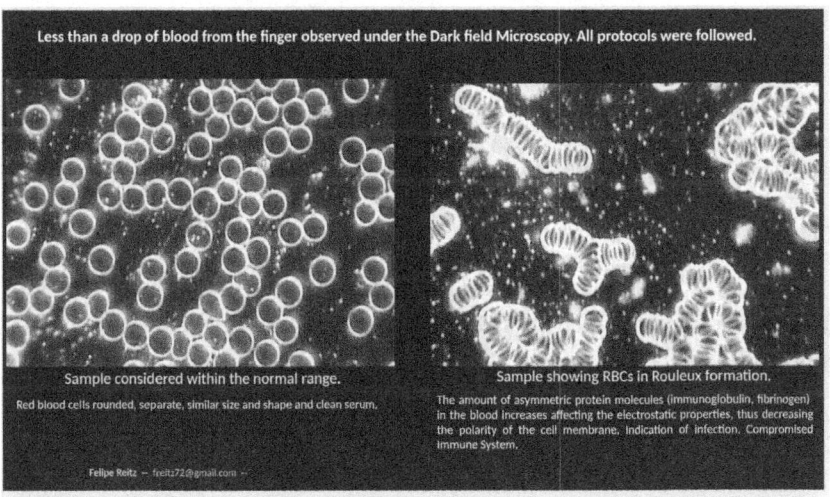

Left: "Red blood cells rounded, separate, similar size and shape and clean serum."
Right: "The amount of asymmetric protein molecules (immunoglobulin, fibrinogen) in the blood increases affecting the electrostatic properties, thus decreasing the polarity of the cell membrane. Indication of infection. Compromised Immune System."

[551] As presented by Dr. Jane Ruby in an interview by Stew Peters (Aug. 19, 2021). https://www.europereloaded.com/vaxxed-blood-shows-stacking-typical-of-blood-cancer/

[552] Dr. Zandré Botha interviewed by Stew Peters, https://rumble.com/vnbgal-never-before-seen-blood-doctor-reveals-horrific-findings-after-examining-vi.html (Oct 4, 2021).

[553] Dr. Ryan Cole interviewed by Greg Hunter, https://usawatchdog.com/global-cv19-vax-absolute-insanity-dr-ryan-cole/ (June 4, 2022)

[554] Franco Giovannini, MD, Riccardo Benzi Cipelli, MD, DDS, and Gianpaolo Pisano, MD, OHNS. Dark -Field Microscopic Analysis on the Blood of 1,006 Symptomatic Persons After Anti-COVID mRNA Injections from Pfizer/BioNtech or Moderna. IJVTPR *2*(2), August 12, 2022 Page | 385. https://ijvtpr.com/index.php/IJVTPR/article/view/47 (Aug. 12, 2022); reported in *The Epoch Times* article: Enrico Trigoso, https://www.theepochtimes.com/foreign-metal-like-objects-some-appearing-as-graphene-family-superstructures-found-in-94-percent-of-people-who-took-mrna-vaccines-italian-doctors_4702330.html (Sept. 6, 2022)

[555] Young Mi Lee MD, Sunyoung Park MD, PhD, IBCLC,and Ki-Yeob Jeon MD, PhD, ScD. "Foreign Materials in Blood Samples of Recipients of COVID-19 Vaccines," https://ijvtpr.com/index.php/IJVTPR/article/view/37 (March 11, 2022)

[556] Felipe Reitz, "My Findings and Observations with Peripheral Live Blood Analysis And Computerized Thermographic Imaging." https://www.documentcloud.org/documents/22275554-epoch-times-info-enrico

[557] Enrico Trigoso, https://www.theepochtimes.com/foreign-metal-like-objects-some-appearing-as-graphene-family-superstructures-found-in-94-percent-of-people-who-took-mrna-vaccines-italian-doctors_4702330.html (Sept. 6, 2022)

[558] The German Working Group for COVID Vaccine Analysis, "Summary of Preliminary Findings," https://s3.documentcloud.org/documents/22140176/report-from-working-group-of-vaccine-analysis-in-germany.pdf (06.07.2022)

[559] Young Mi Lee MD, Sunyoung Park MD, PhD, IBCLC,and Ki-Yeob Jeon MD, PhD, ScD. "Foreign Materials in Blood Samples of Recipients of COVID-19 Vaccines," https://ijvtpr.com/index.php/IJVTPR/article/view/37 (March 11, 2022)

[560] "Australian Whistleblower Scientists Provide Evidence of Nanotech & Graphene Oxide," https://zeeemedia.com/interview/exclusive-australian-whistleblower-scientists-provide-evidence/ (April 3, 2022).

[561] Dr. Zandré Botha interviewed by Stew Peters, https://rumble.com/vnbgal-never-before-seen-blood-doctor-reveals-horrific-findings-after-examining-vi.html (Oct 4, 2021).

[562] Id.

[563] Franco Giovannini, MD, Riccardo Benzi Cipelli, MD, DDS, and Gianpaolo Pisano, MD, OHNS. Dark -Field Microscopic Analysis on the Blood of 1,006 Symptomatic Persons (cited above)

[564] Felipe Reitz, "My Findings and Observations with Peripheral Live Blood Analysis And Computerized Thermographic Imaging." (cited above)

Chapter 39
Dangers of Certain Disclosed Ingredients

Even some of the disclosed ingredients raise serious toxicity issues. Now that new formulations of the vaccines are being distributed, the lists of ingredients should be compared with the lists for the original formulations to check for any differences. The lists of ingredients for the Pfizer, Moderna, Johnson & Johnson and the new Novavax vaccines can be found on the CDC website. [565]

One of the physicians who has addressed the topic of some of the disclosed ingredients from the original formulations is LTC Theresa Long, MD, one of the military doctor whistleblowers cited in Part 2. She submitted a sworn affidavit in the Robert v. Austin case with her findings and conclusions, along with extensive supporting documentation.[566] Other sworn affidavits concerning the dangers of some of the disclosed ingredients, made by Dr. Ralph Grams, MD and another military whistleblower, MAJ Sam Sigoloff, D.O., are included in the same extensive document as LTC Long's affidavit.

First, Dr. Long noted that the label for Comirnaty and BioNTech (both Pfizer products) states that the shots should not be given to people with allergies to any ingredients. *Are people being asked about allergies before being given the shots?* Most people probably do not know if they are allergic to certain ingredients or not. In particular, LTC Long reported her concern about the ingredient *polyethylene glycol*, or PEG. Based on her research, 72% of the population already has PEG antibodies, and people who are allergic to PEG may suffer a severe anaphylactic response resulting in hospitalization or even death.

A paper entitled "A Cautionary Note: Toxicity of Polyethylene Glycol 200 injected intraperitoneally into mice," demonstrates that the route of exposure to a particular chemical matters.[567] In other words, as explained by Dr. Deborah Viglione, substances that may be safe enough to be ingested can be toxic or lethal if injected intramuscularly or intravenously. As stated in the Abstract of that report: "although PEG 200 is generally considered to be harmless it can be toxic when injected i.p. [intraperitoneally]." Half of the research animals in that study had to be euthanized. Therefore, the route of exposure or the manner in which a chemical is taken into the body can have a significant difference in its effects.

Another primary ingredient Dr. Long noted in Pfizer's lipid nanoparticles is ALC 0315. The toxicity report on that ingredient, which she said comprises 30-50% of the total ingredients, says that it is "Category 2 under the OSHA HCS regulations, 21 CFR 1910." It includes several concerning warnings, including but not limited to "seeking medical attention if it comes into contact with your skin…" Most concerning of all, it states: "the chemical, physical and toxicological properties have not been completely investigated" and ends with the caution: **"Product has not been fully validated for medical applications. For research use only."** Dr. Long's conclusion was:

> "due to the risk associated with the spike proteins themselves, due to the risk associated with the lipid nanoparticles (ALC 0315) and adjuvants such as PEG, I believe it is reasonable to conclude that these shots pose a serious risk to many humans due to direct adverse effect or allergic reaction, and therefore should not take vaccinations with either Comirnaty or BioNTech."

She also stated: "My assessment is that ALC 0315 is a known toxin with little study, specifically it is still lacking toxicity, carcinogenic, and teratogenic studies and is specifically restricted to 'research only.'"

LTC Long also studied the safety data for Moderna's SM-102 and stated in her affidavit: "Suffice it to say that SM-102 is significantly more dangerous than the Pfizer ALC 0135…" She noted that the DOD was not at that time actively acquiring or distributing the Moderna product, but stated that if they did:

> "one can expect a much higher Serious Adverse Event and fatality rate given that SM-102 carries an express warning "Skull and Crossbones" characterized under the GHS06 and GHS08. In other words, the Moderna ingredient is deadly."

DANGERS OF CERTAIN DISCLOSED INGREDIENTS

The website of a company called Cayman Chemical [568] contains the following statements on its safety data sheet for SM-102: "This product is for research use - Not for human or veterinary diagnostic or therapeutic use." One of the hazards is listed as "harmful if swallowed." ***Why would Moderna include such a chemical in these shots, and how did the FDA allow an ingredient with these kinds of warnings?***

---

[565] https://www.cdc.gov/coronavirus/2019-ncov/vaccines/different-vaccines/overview-COVID-19-vaccines.html

[566] Affidavit of LTC. Theresa Long, MD in Support of a Motion for a Preliminary Injunction in the case of Robert v. Austin et al, filed in the Federal District Court for the District of Colorado. Civil Action No. 1:21-cv-002228, Sept 24, 2021; https://www.courtlistener.com/docket/60219585/17/robert-v-austin/. Affidavits of MAJ Sam Sigoloff, D.O., and Dr. Ralph Grams, MD, start at pages 41 and 228, respectively.

[567] Thiele W, Kyjacova L, Köhler A, Sleeman JP. A cautionary note: Toxicity of polyethylene glycol 200 injected intraperitoneally into mice. Lab Anim. 2020 Aug;54(4):391-396. doi: 10.1177/0023677219873684. Epub 2019 Sep 16. PMID: 31526095. https://pubmed.ncbi.nlm.nih.gov/31526095/

[568] https://cdn.caymanchem.com/cdn/msds/33474m.pdf

The affidavits of the three doctors mentioned above are accessible at the link provided in the above endnote, or via the following QR Code or at SallySaxon.com:

Chapter 40
Undisclosed Substances – General Concerns

As a backdrop to a brief discussion of two main undisclosed substances reported by researchers who have examined contents of the vaccine vials, it is helpful to first connect certain other dots about some things we already know that provide an important context for what we do not know.

We already know about the elites' desire to control the entire world, including every aspect of every person's life. We have experienced various kinds of authoritarian controls already during COVID, such as lockdowns, mask and vaccine mandates, social distancing, "tracking" and "vaccine passports." We know their keen interest in gathering as much data on us as they can. We have also seen their intention to fuse technology and the human body and to use gene editing. We have evidence of the potential for the COVID shots to change DNA and the elites' interest in "hacking" DNA, the "software of life," even to change what it means to be human.

We also know that Moderna has partnered with a company to use Moderna's mRNA technology for gene editing. Pfizer has also shown that it is pursuing gene-editing technology. Moderna has described its mRNA technology as being like an "operating system" in a computer that can "plug and play" the "software of life," DNA. We know that the government and the manufacturers have advised people to get multiple shots of the COVID "vaccine," even within one year's time, with no apparent end in sight. There are many other relevant facts you may recall from earlier in this book.

Discussion of the researchers' findings gets into some issues that are not traditional medical issues, so most physicians and other health care professionals may not be familiar with them. But because they involve potentially significant safety and health concerns, it is important to be aware of them. Examples of such unfamiliar issues would be the various technologies discussed above and the role of mRNA and nanotechnology in such uses and other biomedical applications. Because of the serious issues raised by the researchers' findings and conclusions, we believe it would be wise for the medical community not to ignore or dismiss them, unless and until there are clear and properly done studies revealing there is no real cause for concern. However, at the present time, there is enough evidence that merits further research by experts in several scientific and medical disciplines to determine the safety and possible health impacts of these new "vaccines."

This is especially important in light of the fact that new formulations of COVID vaccines under the "Future Framework," first administered in September 2022, *do not have to go through any new clinical trials. What do we actually know about what the FDA is requiring of the manufacturers for these new formulations under this new framework? Is any safety testing of any kind being done on new formulations, or are the regulators and the manufacturers looking for safety signals only after their release into the marketplace (if at all)?* Given that researchers have found a variety of undisclosed substances in the original formulations that *did* go through some semblance of regulatory review and clinical trials, there are very good reasons to be highly concerned about what could be in the new formulations that require no such review. There is too much we do not know at this point.

The Main Undisclosed Substances.

Researchers from several different countries have used various kinds of microscopes and imaging equipment to examine the contents of many COVID vaccine vials. They are from Spain,[569] New Zealand,[570] Australia,[571] Germany and Austria,[572] U.S.,[573] UK,[574] South Korea,[575] Argentina,[576] and other countries. They have looked at samples made by Pfizer, Moderna, Johnson & Johnson, AstraZeneca and other companies. Analyses of their findings have revealed very disturbing results. There are various kinds of undisclosed substances you should be aware of that researchers have reported to be in vials from all of those companies (although not all researchers have examined vials from all companies). This report will briefly discuss two main kinds: 1) "foreign or strange objects or structures" and 2) forms of graphene, such as graphene oxide ("GO"), graphene hydroxide, or reduced graphene oxide.

Other possible undisclosed substances: *Are there any other undisclosed materials inside the lipid nanoparticles? Anything that might cause disease, disable the immune system, or change DNA?* We know the mRNA is carrying instructions, but instructions to *do what*? Supposedly the instructions are to make spike protein, *but is there anything else?* According to Dr. Paul Marik, MD, the mRNA in the shots is not a direct copy of the mRNA in SARS-CoV-2. He says it has been genetically altered, so we do not know what it was designed to do or may do unintentionally.[577]

---

[569] Prof. Dr. Pablo Campra, of the Universidad de Almeria, "Detection of Graphene in COVID19 Vaccines by Micro-Raman Spectroscopy: Technical Report,"https://foreignaffairsintelligencecouncil.files.wordpress.com/2021/11/detection-of-graphene-in-covid-19-vaccines-under-micro-raman-spectroscopy.pdf (Nov. 2, 2021)

[570] Dr. Robin Wakeling,Ph.D.. https://odyssee.com/@drsambailey:c/nz-scientist-examines-pfizer-jab-under-the-microscope:6 (March 24 2022)

[571] Presented by Maria Zeee on behalf of Australian scientists, www.seeemedia.com, "Australian Whistleblower Scientists Provide Evidence of Nanotech & Graphene Oxide," https://zeeemedia.com/interview/exclusive-australian-whistleblower-scientists-provide-evidence/ (April 3, 2022)

[572] German and Austrian doctors: https://freedomstrike.org/2021/09/22/german-pathologists-call-for-covid-vaxx-suspension/ (Sept. 22, 2021); and the transcript at https://freedomstrike.org/2021/09/22/german-pathologists-call-for-covid-vaxx-suspension-english-transcript/

[573] Dr. Robert O. Young, https://www.drrobertyoung.com/post/transmission-electron-microscopy-reveals-graphene-oxide-in-cov-19-vaccines (Feb. 5, 2021, updated Oct. 1, 2021 and March 12, 2022)

[574] Project CUNIT-2-112Y6580, "Qualitative Evaluation of Inclusions in Moderna, AstraZeneca and Pfizer COVID-19 vaccines," http://ukcitizen2021.org/Case_Briefing_Document_and_lab_report_Ref_AUC_101_Report%20.pdf

[575] Young Mi Lee MD, Sunyoung Park MD, PhD, IBCLC,and Ki-Yeob Jeon MD, PhD, ScD. "Foreign Materials in Blood Samples of Recipients of COVID-19 Vaccines," https://ijvtpr.com/index.php/IJVTPR/article/view/37/74 (March 11, 2022)

[576] Dr. Martin Monteverde, https://www.orwell.city/2022/01/argentina.html (Jan. 27, 2022)

[577] https://media.mercola.com/ImageServer/Public/2022/June/PDF/post-vaccine-syndrome-protocol-pdf.pdf (June 18, 2022)

Chapter 41
"Strange Objects and Structures"

It is not a secret that the COVID vaccines contain lipid nanoparticles, which are one of many forms of nanotechnology. Their purpose is to carry and deliver the mRNA into the cells. "Nanomedicine" is said to involve "the use of nanoscale materials, such as biocompatible nanoparticles and nanorobots, for diagnosis, delivery, sensing or actuation purposes in a living organism."[578] Nanoparticles are far too small to be seen by the naked eye, or even under a regular or light microscope. "A nanometer is 1/80000th the diameter of an eyelash, one-millionth the size of a pinhead." [579] More powerful and specialized equipment is necessary to see them. For example, Raman spectroscopy is able to "provide a wealth of biochemical information... and achieve high chemical specificity in biological samples." [580] There is quite a large number of reports in the medical and scientific literature about nanotechnology being used in various biomedical applications.

One article is called "Self-assembled mRNA vaccines." [581] It was published right after the COVID vaccine rollout, so many parts of the discussion explained how mRNA vaccines *were supposed to work*. It was too early to address how the shots *actually* worked when administered on a widespread basis, but it still provides helpful explanations of some aspects of the technology. It refers to the COVID-19 vaccines as having "pushed the boundaries of gene therapy," and also explains:

> "Self-assembly of 'smart' materials is a highly sought-after approach in many areas of materials science - simply mix the components, and intermolecular interactions will assemble these components into the desired structure with the desired properties ... The use of self-assembly has found applications in numerous fields of nanoscience, including nanomedicine. In gene delivery, building blocks such as small molecules or polymers interact with nucleic acids and self-assemble into ordered structures."

The developments in nanomedicine, the acknowledged use of nanotechnology in the mRNA vaccines, and the "self-assembly" feature of nanomaterials all put the findings of those who have examined COVID vaccine vials in a different light than they might otherwise have appeared. The COVID vaccine researchers from around the world report finding various kinds of "strange objects and structures," things they have never seen before. Some appear as strange crystals, others as "folded ribbons," while others are "self-assembling" structures that resemble electronic circuitry like a router with antennae. The circuity-like structures are apparently not seen immediately when a drop from the vials is put under a microscope. The self-assembly process appears to occur over a period of time.

As one would expect, those promoting the vaccines as safe and effective have denied such findings and have sought to discredit the researchers who have reported them. Some have claimed that a chip for tracking and other purposes is too big to fit inside a syringe.[582] Technically that is true with regard to pre-assembled chips, but they ignore or fail to acknowledge the existence of *self-assembling nanotechnology*. Since a picture is worth a thousand words, some of the photos taken of what researchers are reporting to have seen using various kinds of specialized microscopic equipment may help many decide what to believe about this subject.

Figures 8 to 17 below show some of the various kinds of objects found by researchers who have examined the contents of COVID vaccine vials from various manufacturers, including some self-assembled structures. Not every vial contains all the same kinds of objects. In addition to the sample photos below, others are available in various other studies and independent media sources, such as Australian investigative journalist, Maria Zeee;[583] a UK research group,[584] Dr. Martin Monteverde of Argentina,[585] and http://LifeoftheBlood.com.

Figures 8 (below, left) **and 9** (below, right), as well as **Figures 10 and 11** are from the Conference of German and Austrian Doctors held in December 2021.[586] According to the researchers, these photos are of the same object, but Fig. 9 shows what the object in Fig. 8 developed into 3 months later (starting at about the 1:30:40 mark in the video). This is from a Pfizer/BioNTech vial. Notice the general similarities between Figure 9 here and Figure 12 below. Though the detail in Figure 9 is difficult to see because of the dark background, if these two images in Figures 8 and 9 are of the same object at different points in time, it is very clear that the simpler object on the left has developed into something quite different.

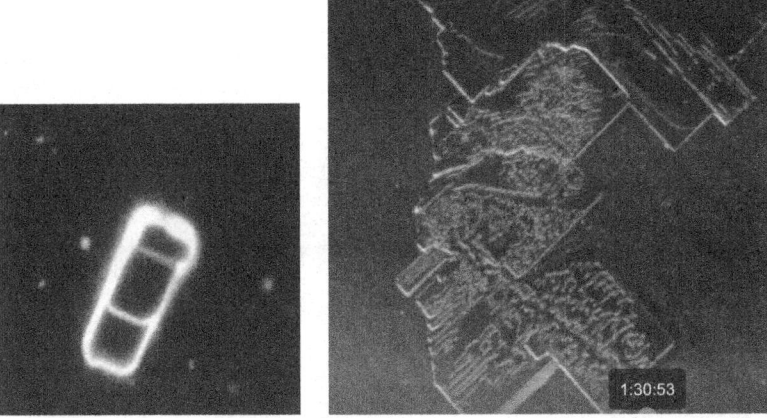

Figures 10 (left) and 11 (right)[587] at the 1:48:41 mark in the video. **Figure 11** appears to be the same as Figure 10, except that it is not illuminated and is slightly larger, allowing somewhat more detail to be observed.

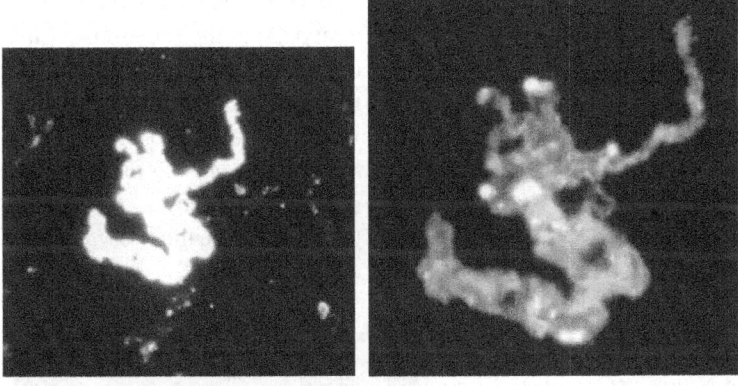

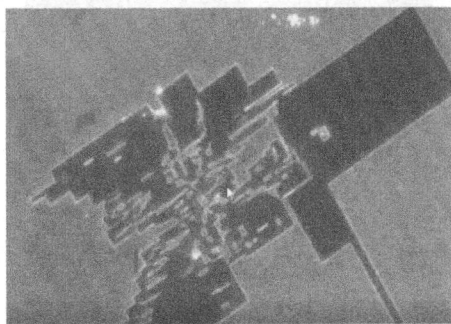

Figure 12 [588] is a photo from www.LifeoftheBlood.com that was used in a presentation by Dr. Robin Wakeling (New Zealand). It depicts more clearly a structure or object similar to the one shown in Figure 9 above.

Figures 13-15 [589] are from The German Working Group for COVID Vaccine Analysis, Summary of Preliminary Findings.

Figures 13 (left) and 14 (right) – at p. 14 of their report, are from a Johnson & Johnson vial. The legend in the original photo states: "It should be noted that objects of this type were not found in all of the samples."

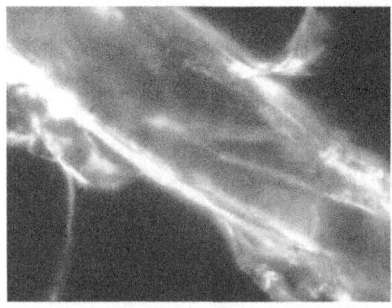 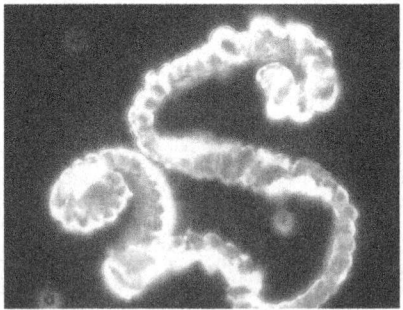

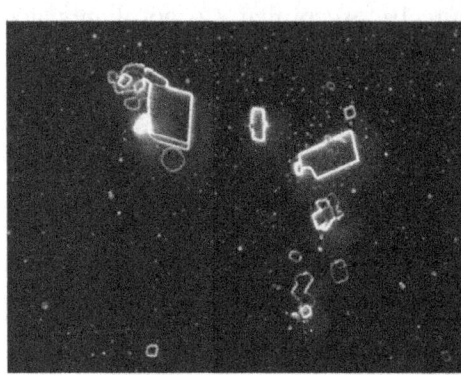

Figure 15.[590] The original description by the German Working Group for their Figure 4 on p. 24 of their report is: "Lipid crystal particles at 1,000x magnification in the Comirnaty vaccine from BioNTech/Pfizer. Some of the crystals are in the size range of red blood cells (Ø 7-8 µm], the so-called erythrocytes and even larger."

Figure 16. [591] Photo provided by Dr. Daniel Nagase (Canada) of one drop from a Pfizer vial using an electron microscope. In one droplet he said there are hundreds of these little squares.

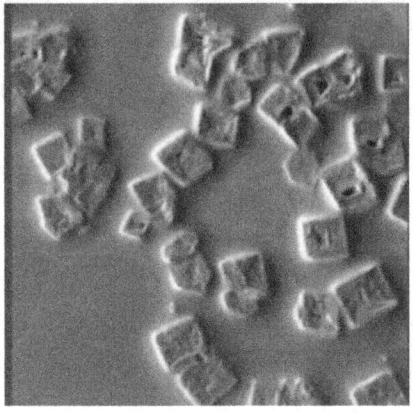

STRANGE OBJECTS AND STRUCTURES

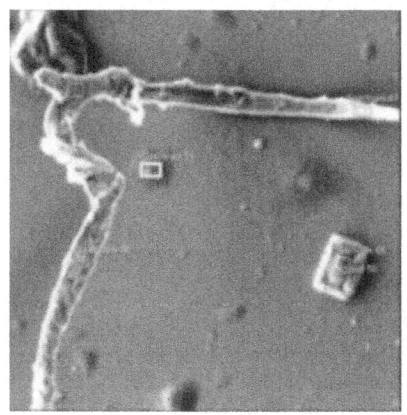

Figure 17. [592] This is another photo provided by Dr. Daniel Nagase from a Pfizer sample using an electron microscope. It shows some kind of fiber-like object in addition to squares and other objects. He also said that "the x-ray diffraction spectroscopy of the squares and fibre showed mostly Carbon and Oxygen."

What are these strange objects and what is their purpose? What do they have to do with protecting a person from infection or disease? In light of statements by Klaus Schwab and Yuval Noah Harari, especially Harari's statement about COVID being remembered as the time when "surveillance went under the skin," consider the following explanation about the possible purpose of these foreign objects. In an article entitled "How it All Fits Together: Covid, 5G, Nanotech, Transhumanism and Charles Lieber," Maryam Henein states:

> "The wireless future is here. The model ostensibly turns human beings, via nano-implants, into antennas that can transmit information. They're turning human beings into quasi-machines. Under this transhumanist agenda, the idea is to place nanotech inside our bodies [so that] we can communicate in real-time with the Smart Grid powered by way of 5G.
>
> "It's called the 'internet of bodies' (IoB) or the 'nanotech of things,' (NToT), and it connects with the Internet of Things (IOT). One way this is accomplished is to embed graphene-made sensors into fabrics. Another is to implant or ingest the nanotech matter into the body, creating an internal technology platform." [593]

Internal technology platform? Does that not sound like Moderna's earlier description of its mRNA technology? How about Harari's statements about "hacking humans?" Are the pieces of the puzzle starting to fall into place? Readers who would like to take a deeper dive into these

251

issues may want to consider Karen Kingston's outstanding research referred to earlier.[594]

---

[578] https://www.nature.com/subjects/nanomedicine

[579] Maryam Henein, https://truthcomestolight.com/how-it-all-fits-together-covid-5g-nanotech-transhumanism-charles-lieber/ (Feb 6, 2022)

[580] https://microscopy.arizona.edu/event/bio-raman-aug2019

[581] Kim J, Eygeris Y, Gupta M, Sahay G. Self-assembled mRNA vaccines. Adv Drug Deliv Rev. 2021 Mar;170:83-112. doi: 10.1016/j.addr.2020.12.014. Epub 2021 Jan 2. PMID: 33400957; PMCID: PMC7837307. https://pubmed.ncbi.nlm.nih.gov/33400957

[582] Katie Schoolov, https://www.cnbc.com/2021/10/01/why-the-covid-vaccines-dont-contain-a-magnetic-5g-tracking-chip.html (Oct. 1, 2021)

[583] "Australian Whistleblower Scientists Provide Evidence of Nanotech & Graphene Oxide," https://zeeemedia.com/interview/exclusive-australian-whistleblower-scientists-provide-evidence/ (April 3, 2022)

[584] https://worldcouncilforhealth.org/multimedia/covid-19-vaccines-contents-prelim-summary-rob-verkerk. The lab research was done by a group called EbMCsquared.

[585] Dr, Martin Monteverde presentation, https://www.orwell.city/2022/01/argentina.html

[586] Conference of German and Austrian Doctors, https://odysee.com/@en:a5/PK_Tot-durch-Impfung_english:a (Dec. 4, 2021)

[587] Id.

[588] This photo is from www.LifeoftheBlood.com as presented by Dr. Robin Wakeling, https://odysee.com/@drsambailey:c/nz-scientist-examines-pfizer-jab-under-the-microscope:6 (March 22, 2022)

[589] The German Working Group for COVID Vaccine Analysis, Summary of Preliminary Findings. https://s3.documentcloud.org/documents/22140176/report-from-working-group-of-vaccine-analysis-in-germany.pdf, (06.07.2022)

[590] Id.

[591] Personal communication between Dr. Daniel Nagase and James Thorp, MD, Nov. 2022; Dr. Daniel Nagase interviewed by Melanie Risdon, https://rumble.com/v11go0d-watch-dr.-nagase-reviews-images-from-covid-vaccines-shows-no-elements-of-li.html (April 18, 2022); Transcript of interview of Dr. Daniel Nagase with Melanie Risdon in the previous reference: https://expose-news.com/wp-content/uploads/2022/05/Transcript-Dr.-Daniel-Nagase.pdf (April 18, 2022)

[592] Personal communication between Dr. Daniel Nagase and James Thorp, MD, Nov. 2022; Dr. Daniel Nagase interviewed by Melanie Risdon (cited above)

[593] Maryam Henein, https://truthcomoestolight.com/how-it-all-fits-together-covid-5g-nanotech-transhumanism-charles-lieber/ (Feb, 6, 2022)

[594] http://karenkingston.substack.com/ ; https://citizens.news/663687.html (Oct. 6, 2022)

Chapter 42
Graphene – Is it in the COVID "Vaccines?"

If graphene oxide or other forms of graphene had been identified by only one or two researchers as being in the COVID vaccine vials, there would be reason to be skeptical. However, when many researchers, such as those whose photos are presented above and others, in many different countries, working independently and using various kinds of microscopes, all find basically the same or similar things, their findings merit deeper consideration. This is especially the case when the medical and scientific literature in recent years show that a very large number of papers have been published on the subject of the great advantages of using graphene oxide for drug delivery and even in mRNA products.[595] Not surprisingly, "fact-checkers" and those promoting the official narrative deny that there is graphene in the COVID shots.

Graphene has been called a "supermaterial" because it is "200x stronger than steel by weight, 1,000x lighter than paper, 98% transparent, conducts electricity better than any other known material at room temperature, it can convert light at any wavelength into a current, and it is made from carbon, the fourth most abundant element in the universe..."[596] No wonder Prof. A. Fasano, Co-Director of the Surgical Program for Movement Disorders at Toronto University Hospital, said in 2018 that *"Graphene is the next big thing in bioengineering materials ..."*[597] It enables "interface with the nervous system, allegedly with fewer side effects than other materials."[598]

The main form of graphene found by the independent researchers is graphene oxide,[599] though other forms have also been reported. However, they all claim that graphene in its various forms is toxic. *If that is true, why has it become a highly favored substance for use in biomedical applications? Therefore, the questions are: 1) is graphene oxide (or other form of graphene) actually in the COVID vaccines? 2) if so, for what purpose? and 3) is it toxic, and if so, can its toxicity be sufficiently mediated?*

Evidence that graphene oxide is in the shots

There are various kinds of evidence that reveal the presence of some form of graphene in the shots. Prof. Dr. Pablo Campra of the Universidad de Almeria, Spain, was the first to issue an interim report on graphene-related materials in the COVID vaccines in June 2021. He issued a later report in November 2021.[600] Using micro-Raman spectroscopy, he screened more than 110 objects for their "graphene-like appearance" under optical microscopy. He chose 28, of which 8 had a conclusive identification of "graphene oxide structure" and the other 20 objects "show a very high level of compatibility with undetermined graphene structures."

An interim study reported in February 2022 by *The Exposé*[601] was a forensic analysis by a UK lab investigating COVID vaccine vials to verify Dr. Campra's findings and report any other ingredients that might be toxic to the body.[602] The UK lab examined two vials of Moderna and one each of Pfizer and AstraZeneca. Raman spectroscopy was the chosen method for initial identification, but other microscopy was also used. The Executive Summary states that their initial findings "confirm the presence of graphene compounds in each of the injection vials."

They also identified five basic kinds of various graphene-based forms: ribbons (coated with polyethylene glycol), sheet forms, tubular forms, nano dots and nano scrolls. That could account for the different shapes and sizes of the objects in the above photos. All three vaccines in the UK study used "self-assembling lipid nano particles as drug delivery mechanisms." They concluded by saying that the four samples "all contain significant amounts of carbon composites, graphene compounds and iron oxide," and were not disclosed by the manufacturers. They described as "striking" the percentage of the ingredients consisting of graphene and other carbon composites. However, they also noted the increasing use of graphene in drug delivery which should be considered. ***But that does not excuse the manufacturers from not disclosing it, nor does it explain why the manufacturers would hide the inclusion of graphene-family nanoparticles in the vaccines from the public.***

Dr. Daniel Nagase is another doctor who has examined Pfizer and Moderna vials.[603] Two of his photos of foreign objects are shown above. The vials he received had been unrefrigerated for one to two months. He examined the contents under an electron microscope which enabled him to determine the chemical composition of the contents. His analysis showed that by far the predominant element in the objects was carbon, and graphene is made of carbon atoms. Different objects had a smattering of various other elements, but they were not all the same, even in objects in the same drop. However, there was no nitrogen or phosphorous, which, he explained, means that the objects were not biologic in nature; otherwise, they would have nitrogen and phosphorous.

Other evidence of graphene in the vaccines comes from Argentina where it was reported in January, 2022, that a public health official, Dr. Patricia Aprea, admitted in a court case that the COVID vaccines administered there do contain graphene.[604] The case involved a death following a COVID vaccination, but the report did not specify which manufacturer's vaccine was involved.

Karen Kingston has uncovered documentary evidence of it being in the COVID-19 vaccines, or at least some of them.[605] As stated earlier, she has extensive knowledge about the COVID vaccines, the serious problems with the clinical trials and the contents of many relevant documents of the manufacturers and the regulatory agencies. Kingston says that graphene is not mentioned in the U.S. vaccine patents, but points to a patent application that was filed in China in 2020 by the Shanghai Engineering Research Center for Nanotechnology.[606] That document states that it "relates to a vaccine:"

> "…in particular to development of a 2019-nCoV coronavirus nuclear recombinant nano vaccine ... The novel coronavirus vaccine contains **graphene oxide**, carnosine, CpG and novel coronavirus RBD; The carnosine, the CpG and novel coronavirus RBD are combined on a framework of the **graphene oxide**…" (emphasis added)

Purpose: *Why would graphene oxide be in a "vaccine"?*

There are at least a couple purposes graphene oxide could serve in the COVID shots. One is that graphene oxide plays an important role in self-assembly, which would explain the self-assembly described by the researchers during their microscopic examinations. This is explained in an article entitled "New graphene-based material self-assembles into vascular structures":

> "Self-assembly is the process by which multiple components spontaneously organize into larger, well-defined structures. Biological systems rely on this process to controllably assemble molecular building blocks ... to grow, replicate and perform robust functions.
>
> "The new biomaterial is produced by the self-assembly of a protein with graphene oxide. This self-assembly process allows the flexible (disordered) regions of the protein to order and conform to the graphene oxide, generating a strong interaction between them. By controlling the way in which the two components are mixed, it is possible to guide their assembly at multiple scales in the presence of cells to produce complex robust structures." [607]

Another very important purpose for using graphene would be its excellent electrical conductivity properties in connection with the "foreign objects" found in the vials. If some or all of those objects are in fact some kind of nanotechnology designed to provide connection to an external server, as suggested by their appearance, the article by Maryam Henein quoted above does indeed provide a logical explanation as to "How it All Fits Together," as the title of her article suggests. She explains that graphene is necessary for the connectivity to occur. The 5G acts upon the graphene. That interaction of 5G and graphene is discussed further below in the section on 5G. Henein also points out that this area of nanotechnology is totally unregulated, so we need to be all the more vigilant about what we put into our bodies.

In an article entitled "Graphene Oxide. & Nano-Router Circuitry in Covid Vaccines: Uncovering the True Purpose of These Mandatory Toxic Injections," author Mik Anderson states:[608]

> "The properties of graphene are exceptional from the physical point of view, but also thermodynamic, electronic, mechanical and magnetic. Its characteristics allow its use as a superconductor, electromagnetic wave absorbing material (microwave EM), emitter, signal receiver, quantum antenna, which makes it possible to create advanced electronics on a nano and micrometric scale...
>
> Second, graphene is a radio-modulable nanomaterial, capable of absorbing electromagnetic waves and multiplying radiation, acting as a nano-antenna, or a signal repeater."

GRAPHENE – IS IT IN THE COVID VACCINES?

That article cites many references related to this topic. *As the title of that article and the article on "How it all Fits Together" suggest, is this technology the real purpose behind the COVID "vaccines"? Are the pieces of the puzzle starting to come together to enable us to see where and how "all things COVID" fit into the "big picture" discussed at the beginning of this Part 4?*

Toxicity of Graphene

There is a large number of studies that address the issue of toxicity of graphene oxide (GO) in the human body. One such paper is entitled "Synthesis and Toxicity of Graphene Oxide Nanoparticles: A Literature Review of In Vitro and In Vivo Studies" published in 2021.[609] Based upon those authors' extensive review of the existing literature, they noted that the studies on graphene oxide's cytotoxicity were contradictory. To complicate the matter, they also found that the "dependence of cytotoxicity on dose changes with different cell types." Their conclusion was:

> "Although GO is useful for many applications, there is still a risk related to its 'toxicity,' limiting its uses. Studies conducted so far indicate that the toxicity of GO could depend on its size, synthesis methods, route of administration, and exposure time. In addition, we presented the different toxic effects of this nanomaterial at the cellular and systemic level of the body with discussions on the underlying toxicological mechanism. We also highlighted the role of biological barriers to the entry of GO into the body and its toxicokinetics. ROS-mediated cellular damage has been postulated as a primary mechanism of GO cytotoxicity. In general, available GO toxicity studies are mainly limited to evaluating acute toxicity, while chronic toxicological studies lack."

Another paper published in November 2020 cautioned that preclinical studies to date were not adequate. It stated that most studies about graphene-based nanoparticles were focused more on "delivering their burden in the body" with only scarce attention paid to their removal. The paper also said that the main toxicity issue is "interaction between graphene nanomaterials and cells/tissues..."[610] It concluded:

> "Although many efforts have been made to reduce the toxicity of the graphene and graphene-based materials, the use of these

compounds is currently associated with high risk. Recently, these materials were put into the list of hazardous agents by The European Scientific Committee on Emerging and Newly Identified Health Risks (SCENIHR).[198]" [footnote in original]

Some of the problems resulting from GO toxicity are discussed in a 2016 paper entitled "Toxicity of graphene-family nanoparticles: a general review of the origins and mechanisms." [611] They "can induce acute and chronic injuries in tissues by penetrating through the blood-air barrier, blood-testis barrier, blood-brain barrier, and blood-placenta barrier etc. and accumulating in the lung, liver, and spleen etc... granulomas, lung fibrosis …inflammatory response … autophagy and necrosis." Cytotoxicity in vitro has also been verified to "change the cell viability and morphology, destroy membrane integrity, and induce DNA damage, … decrease cell adhesion; induce cell apoptosis; and enter lysosomes, mitochondria, cell nuclei, and endoplasm; GQDs entered cells and induced DNA damage by increased expression of p53, Rad51, and OGG1 proteins in NIH-3 T3 cells." [612] The paper states that there were such "a mass of data demonstrating the toxicity of GFN's [graphene-family nanoparticles] in different organs or systems in animals, so that it is hard to list all the data in this review." [613] That paper also noted that recent research had focused more on application than on toxicity.

To summarize, because of the number of variables that affect toxicity, it appears that cytotoxicity testing needs to specifically focus on each particular application. It is also apparent that the bulk of the research has focused on the potential uses of graphene-based nanoparticles, to the neglect of toxicity issues. Without specific testing for each application, the risks are significant.

Where are the toxicology studies for the COVID vaccines? What is it about the use of graphene oxide (or other form of graphene) in the vaccines that they do not want us to know?

---

[595] For example, see the article and sources cited in Rhoda Wilson, www.expose-news.com/2022/06/22/vaccine-using-graphene-oxide-sheet-like-nanoparticles/ (June 22, 2022)

[596] Dave Roos, https://science.howstuffworks.com/innovation/new-inventions/graphene.htm (Aug. 18,, 2020)

[597] http://inbrain-neuroelectronics.com/

[598] Chloe Kent, "How Inbrain Neuroelectronics develops graphene-based neural implants," https://www.medicaldevice-network.com/analysis/inbrain-neuroelectronics-graphene/ (March 31, 2021)

[599] "Australian Whistleblower Scientists Provide Evidence of Nanotech & Graphene Oxide," https://zeeemedia.com/interview/exclusive-australian-whistleblower-scientists-provide-evidence/ (April 3, 2022)

[600] Prof. Dr. Pablo Campra, Universidad de Almeria, Spain, "Detection of Graphene in COVID19 Vaccines by Micro-Raman Spectroscopy: Technical Report," https://foreignaffairsintelligencecouncil.files.wordpress.com/2021/11/detection-of-graphene-in-covid-19-vaccines-under-micro-raman-spectroscopy.pdf (Nov. 2, 2021)

[601] Patricia Harrity, https://expose-news.com/2022/02/13/uk-lab-confirms-graphene-in-covid-vaccines/ (Feb. 13, 2022)

[602] Project CUNIT-2-112Y6580, "Qualitative Evaluation of Inclusions in Modern, AstraZeneca and Pfizer COVID-19," vaccines, http://ukcitizen2021.org/Case_Briefing_Document_and_lab_report_Ref_AUC_101_Report%20.pdf

[603] Dr. Daniel Nagase interviewed by Melanie Risdon, https://rumble.com/v11go0d-watch-dr.-nagase-reviews-images-from-covid-vaccines-shows-no-elements-of-li.html (April 18, 2022)

[604] https://www.orwell.city/2022/01/ANMAT.html (Jan. 17, 2022)

[605] Karen Kingston interviewed by Doug Billings, https://dougbillings.us/video/dougs-july-29th-interview-with-karen-kingston-re-posted/

[606] https://patentscope.wipo.int/search/en/detail.jsf?docId=CN317065497&tab=NATIONALBIBLIO

[607] *Materials Today,* "New graphene-based material self-assembles into vascular structures ," https://www.materialstoday.com/materials-chemistry/news/new-graphenebased-material-selfassembles/ (March 18, 2020)

[608] Mik Anderson, https://truthcomestolight.com/graphene-oxide-nano-router-circuitry-in-covid-vaccines-uncovering-the-true-purpose-of-these-mandatory-toxic-injections/ (Nov. 2021)

[609] Asmaa Rhazouani, Halima Gamrani, Mounir El Achaby, Khalid Aziz, Lhoucine Gebrati, Md Sahab Uddin, Faissal AZIZ, "Synthesis and Toxicity of Graphene Oxide Nanoparticles: A Literature Review of *In Vitro* and *In Vivo* Studies", *BioMed Research International*, vol. 2021, Article ID 5518999, 19 pages, 2021. https://doi.org/10.1155/2021/5518999

[610] Hoseini-Ghahfarokhi M, Mirkiani S, Mozaffari N, Abdolahi Sadatlu MA, Ghasemi A, Abbaspour S, Akbarian M, Farjadian F, Karimi M. Applications of Graphene and Graphene Oxide in Smart Drug/Gene Delivery: Is the World Still Flat? Int J Nanomedicine. 2020 Nov 27;15:9469-9496. doi: 10.2147/IJN.S265876. PMID: 33281443; PMCID: PMC7710865. https://pubmed.ncbi.nlm.nih.gov/33281443/

[611] Ou, L., Song, B., Liang, H. et al. Toxicity of graphene-family nanoparticles: a general review of the origins and mechanisms. *Part Fibre Toxicol* 13, 57 (2016). https://doi.org/10.1186/s12989-016-0168-y

[612] Ibid., p. 8

[613] Ibid., p. 4-5

Chapter 43
5G Issues

Two issues are addressed here concerning 5G and COVID: 1) how graphene in the vaccines interacts with 5G; and 2) the fact that radiation sickness has the same or similar symptoms as COVID-19.

Connection to the Vaccines. Dr. Rob Verkerk is a scientist on the science and medical committee of the World Council for Health. He has summarized the interim findings of the UK lab mentioned above that studied the contents of various COVID vaccine vials. He has been involved in many nano technological investigations, and has studied the use of graphene in nano electronic devices. In summarizing that lab's findings for its Interim Report, he said:[614]

> "So the people who have suggested there may be a link between 5G or 6G electronic devices and graphene are not barking up a conspiracy theory tree. There is genuine reason to be concerned about the linkage between those two things."

Due to the greater demands and requirements for 5G technology, the industry needed new materials that could serve its purposes. A 2019 study also showed that graphene can be applied to 5G.[615] A 2019 article at Graphene-Investors.com revealed that research was being conducted "to see how graphene's high conductivity and flexible monolayer can support the development of 5G wireless technology."[616] In 2017, the article reported, a Swedish research team had a breakthrough in this area when "they combined terahertz detection with flexible graphene, a 5G mobile device controlled the Internet of Things (IoT)." The article further stated: "With the right resources and work, it's only a matter of time before we can benefit from graphene's incorporation into 5G."

For more about the connection between 5G, COVID-19 and the vaccines, see the "Report on 5G Directed Energy Radiation Emissions in the Context of Nanometal-Contaminated Vaccines that include COVID-19 with

5 G ISSUES

Graphite Ferrous Oxide Antennas" by Mark Steele, especially section III of his report.[617] Steele is a British engineer, inventor, patent writer and weapons research scientist with a materials science background. He states: "Cyber Command USA had been made aware of my expertise and specifically requested my advice with regard to an unusual 5G antenna design deployed across the USA." He says:

> "I have acted as a witness and provided statements in several court cases, exposing the lack of any credible evidence that the 5G light-emitting diode (LED) network and planned neural connection to the 5G grid are safe. This includes nano metamaterial technologies that are contaminating vaccinations, that are not legal or lawful, and that breach a number of international and domestic laws."

Think about that: *"Planned neural connections to the 5G grid," about which he says there is no credible evidence of their safety, including "nanomaterial technologies contaminating vaccinations."* He also states that there is a substance in the vaccines that can be activated using electromagnetic radiation for tracking purposes.[618]

Connection to COVID-19. It is reported that in places where 5G was turned up, more people got sick with COVID-like symptoms, including Wuhan, China in late October 2019, just before the outbreak.[619] *Were they sick with "COVID" or was it radiation sickness, or perhaps something else?*

The report by Rubik and Brown cited in the reference below refers to a "large body of peer reviewed literature, since before World War II, on the biological effects of WCR [wireless communications radiation] that impact many aspects of our health." After reviewing those reports, they found "intersections between the pathophysiology of SARS-CoV-2 and detrimental bioeffects of WCR exposure." In Mark Steele's report quoted above, he confirmed this point: "All of the known coronavirus symptoms can be attributed to ionizing and non-ionizing radiation pollution."[620] Just as the symptoms of the flu are similar to COVID-19, and the PCR test could not tell the difference, it appears possible that some who have suffered symptoms of COVID could actually have been suffering from radiation sickness.

There is much more available on this subject, but again, the purpose here is simply to make you aware of the issues. The danger of 5G is another very big issue that should be investigated and dealt with immediately by local government officials. It is also important for doctors to recognize because it could affect their diagnoses and treatments for people suffering its effects.

---

[614] https://worldcouncilforhealth.org/multimedia/covid-19-vaccines-contents-prelim-summary-rob-verkerk. The lab research was done by a group called EbMCsquared.

[615] Sa'don SNH, Jamaluddin MH, Kamarudin MR, Ahmad F, Yamada Y, Kamardin K, Idris IH. Analysis of Graphene Antenna Properties for 5G Applications. Sensors (Basel). 2019 Nov 6;19(22):4835. doi: 10.3390/s19224835. PMID: 31698830; PMCID: PMC6891658. https://pubmed.ncbi.nlm.nih.gov/31698830/

[616] https://graphene-investors.com/graphene-can-put-the-g-in-5g/ (May 21, 2019)

[617] Mark Steele, https://forlifeonearth.weebly.com/mark-steele-expert-report-on-5g-emissions-in-context-of-nanometal-contaminated-vaccines.html

[618] Ibid., p. 12

[619] Beverly Rubik & Robert R. Brown, "Evidence for a connection between coronavirus disease-19 and exposure to radiofrequency radiation from wireless communications including 5G," https://www.ncbi.nlm.nih.gov/pmc/articles/PMC8580522/ (Sept. 29, 2021)

[620] Mark Steele, https://forlifeonearth.weebly.com/mark-steele-expert-report-on-5g-emissions-in-context-of-nanometal-contaminated-vaccines.html, p. 10

Chapter 44
Reflections on Part 4

What do you think about the morality and ethics, not to mention the legality, of injecting various forms of nanotechnology into people without disclosure or informed consent? This may be one of the most deceptive and evil aspects of COVID's role in the big picture. When the elites talk about "fundamentally changing" humans into hybrid creatures who can be surveilled, tracked and controlled, we now understand better what they mean.

That raises several questions, such as: *If these globalists are not stopped, what kind of genetic manipulations might they be planning for humanity? What are the ramifications of creating new hybrid species? How are they planning to use these technologies in the body to track and control people 24/7?*

The globalist elites' desire to control extends to every part of our lives. It includes control over where we can go, what we can do, where we can live, how much energy we consume, what we can say, and whether we even have access to our funds and financial accounts, as the outspoken doctors have been experiencing problems with recently. Having some kind of device "under the skin" would be ideal, from the elites' perspective, to keep track of our compliance and everything we do. They want the world to have a kind of "social credit system" like China already has. That system determines what degree of benefits and privileges each person may enjoy based on their level of compliance with the elites' mandates and dictates. Noncompliance brings punishments and loss of privileges. Having something "under the skin" that they could monitor or even turn on and off at will to control our access to certain activities or privileges would serve their agenda well.

But it goes further than that. Harari has talked about "hacking our bodies" and "re-engineering" our bodies, brains and minds. They could even monitor and control our thoughts and our feelings. That, in turn, determines what we do and how we do it. Remember, Harari also said "free will is over." They have the technology to take away our ability to think and make choices for ourselves, and to program us to do whatever they want us to do. They now have the ability to create synthetic life in various forms. *Is that the kind of life we want for ourselves and future generations?*

Given the extremely serious potential misuses and abuses of technology available today, where do you draw the line between appropriate advancements in health care and the point where it becomes unethical and recklessly dangerous?

Is it clearer now why the government, the controlled media, and the entire medical industrial complex and other elites have been so determined to get everyone on the planet injected with these shots? Do you also see why they had to demonize and refuse to approve all effective treatment protocols for COVID-19? It should be apparent now why they have ignored all of the glaring warning signals in the VAERS database and why they have lied to us all about "all things COVID."

Chapter 45
This is a War

What we have been witnessing since 2020 is frighteningly similar to the history of the 1930's that led to World War II and the genocide of many tens of millions of people. Unfortunately, as the saying goes, those who do not learn from history are bound to repeat it. It appears that we are repeating what our parents and grandparents vowed should never happen again.

During the rise to power of Adolf Hitler and the Nazi party, censorship and control of the various forms of media and communication were tools used to steer the German people into supporting Nazi ideals and beliefs, not realizing that they were actually enabling and supporting a dictatorship that would ultimately lead to the deaths of millions. After the Nazis came to power in 1933 – *through a legal political process,* **not** *by a military coup d'état* – freedom of speech and press in the German constitution was abolished by various decrees and laws. By 1934, criticism of the Nazi government was illegal. At the time, the Nazis controlled all radio and press such as newspapers and magazines. They also influenced the German people through art, theater, and music. The Nazis literally burned books that countered their narrative, or banned them as "un-German." They went so far as to censor soldiers' letters to their loved ones.

In addition, in 1933, they started a new government department led by Joseph Goebbels called The Reich Ministry of Enlightenment and Propaganda. That department began a massive propaganda campaign glorifying the Nazis and desecrating the Jewish people. They created groups to brainwash the youth such as The Hitler Youth and The League of German Girls. Jewish people eventually had to wear bands with a star on their arms to label them publicly, somewhat akin to the purpose of today's "vaccine passports," except that these "passports" identify the "good people."

The description of Holocaust survivor Vera Sharav during an interview with Reiner Fuellmich [621] is especially revealing as it relates to the health care profession. Many of her comments are also presented in the International Criminal Court Complaint referred to in Part 3. [622]

She spoke about how the Nazis destroyed the "moral norms" and drastically changed and perverted the health care profession and institutions. They used public health as a premise for destroying what she called a "social conscience" and to justify trampling on civil and human rights. She told about how public health policies were motivated by eugenics and became a substitute for doctors being able to put their patients' best interests first. She also explained that the Nazis used fear and intimidation to vilify the Jews as ones who were spreading disease and were therefore a health threat to everyone else. She said it was fear and propaganda that explain why the Germans did not stand up to the Nazis' genocide.

She went on to speak about issues more directly related to the medical profession and the entire medical system in terms that are uncomfortably similar to how many have characterized the profession and system in the era of COVID:

> "Medical mandates are a major step backwards towards a fascist dictatorship and genocide. ...The stark lesson of the Holocaust is that whenever doctors join forces with government and deviate from their personal, professional, clinical commitment to do no harm to the individual, medicine can then be perverted from a healing, humanitarian profession to a murderous apparatus… **What sets the Holocaust apart from all other mass genocides is the pivotal role played by the medical establishment, the entire medical establishment.** Every step of the murderous process was endorsed by the academic and professional medical establishment. Medical doctors and prestigious medical societies and institutions lent the veneer of legitimacy to infanticide, mass murder of civilians."

She went on to describe a Nazi project called T4, about which she said the purpose was get rid of the economic burden presented by those people considered by the government and the doctors to be "worthless eaters." *Does that not sound similar to Yuval Noah Harari's statements about all those "superfluous people"?* T4 also served as a testing ground for various lethal chemicals and pharmaceuticals. Vera said that the ones who benefited financially from the Nazi genocide were "the corporate elite."

Think about what businesses thrived and grew during the COVID lockdowns and which ones shut down. Vera believes that "COVID-19 has exposed eugenics-driven public health policies," and sees it as "a chilling replay of T4." She observed how "people are being conditioned to submit passively to government dictates."

Other parallels of the last few years are strikingly similar, revealing that we, too, have been in a war, but not a war against a virus. We have been subjected to massive and unprecedented censorship by the "untrustworthy" Trusted News Initiative, censoring vital health information even from highly trained and experienced physicians, scientists and other experts worldwide based on the government's own data. We have seen the massive campaign pushing the COVID "vaccines" as safe and effective through multiple media channels and a government-sponsored COVID-19 Community Corps, despite continual and increasingly strong signals of the terrible harm the shots are causing.

We have seen the ostracizing and demonizing of the "unvaccinated" as selfish, stupid and terrible people who are dangerous to society. We have seen revocations of (and threats to revoke) the professional licenses and certifications of doctors who have dared to counter the official narrative. We have seen illegal vaccine mandates, especially for the military, and by large businesses who were pressured by the government to require vaccination and threaten their non-compliant employees with the loss of their jobs. We have seen the denial of medical and religious exemptions. We have seen the imprisonment and inhumane treatment of Americans based on their political views and trumped-up charges. We have seen gestapo-like unlawful and unjustifiable raids on the homes and offices of law-abiding citizens, because of their political views, including a former president of the United States!

The Biden administration's creation of the "Disinformation Governance Board" in the spring of 2022 appears to have been an American version of the Nazi Ministry of Enlightenment and Propaganda. Fortunately, that Board was paused and later ended before it got off the ground. However, the fact that an American government would even consider creating such an entity that would destroy our 1st Amendment freedom of speech should trouble us all, especially when it involves matters of life and death. Even without such a Board, the control of information by the medical industrial complex through the major media has been just as effective as any formal government department. Look how relatively easy it was for them to persuade many tens of millions of Americans to accept masks and mask mandates, social distancing, lockdowns, the claim of no effective treatments, COVID shots, and "vaccine passports." These successes emboldened the elites to push their agenda even harder. So now we have things like newly formulated COVID vaccines authorized *without any clinical trials or ways to ensure their safety.*

Similar to the youth programs in Germany in the 1930's and '40's, programs to brainwash and radicalize our young people are evident in many places. Schools have become "indoctrination centers" for radical ideologies. Movies, TV programs and other entertainment platforms have portrayed traditional American values, traditions and even common-sense facts as evils that must be eradicated from society, and replaced with dangerous and nonsensical policies, even ones that turn science on its head.

The Nazis' rise to power culminated in WWII which started in 1939 and ended in 1945. The estimated worldwide death count from WWII is around 75 million people. There are no accurate figures as to what the total death count was from the "Jewish" holocaust, but it is estimated at well over 18 million, according to the *Holocaust Encyclopedia.* It is similarly impossible to know how many people have already died due to the COVID vaccines, or how many will die after new boosters. In the next few years, what might others experience due to damage to their immune systems that has unleashed cancers, as well as autoimmune, neurodegenerative, cardiovascular and other diseases? *Could the death toll ultimately surpass the holocaust of WWII?*

But those who received the shots should not despair. God is our ultimate Healer. Nothing is impossible for God.

On the surface, the war we have been in is a war against the creators and promoters of what, in essence, is a man-made biological "weapon" disguised as a virus, and another disguised as a "vaccine" offered as a solution to their self-made crisis. **It is a war against humanity.** That is reflected in the globalists' agenda and worldview articulated by Klaus Schwab and his close advisor, Yuval Noah Harari.

At its root, this is a war in the spiritual realm, a war between good and evil. The wealthy elites are literally trying to "play God" by fundamentally changing what it means to be human. They seek to take technology to its extremes, and to replace *homo sapiens* with "hybrids" and synthetic forms of life using artificial intelligence. The statements by

Schwab and Harari reveal that the elites' agenda goes even further: *they also reject the sanctity of life and the premise that every human life has a divine purpose.* **Their minds and consciences have become so seared by evil that letting people die or even killing them is acceptable, if not also necessary, to achieve their warped objectives.** In their worldview, ridding the population of billions of those they consider "superfluous people" is a desirable objective, just as Vera Sharav said of the Nazis. That explains why they could not care less how many people die and millions of families are devastated by their sinister schemes. *Is that not evil?* **Such is the war that we are fighting.**

This is why many physicians, scientists, attorneys and other experts have characterized the vaccine campaign as *crimes against humanity and genocide, and why they have been willing to risk everything to fight this war for freedom and truth. Why are they not intimidated by the governing medical boards?* I can only speak for Dr. Deborah Viglione and Dr. James Thorp, but besides the fact that they believe freedom and truth are worth fighting for, they also understand their Constitutional and other legal rights. If the governing medical boards were to revoke their licenses and other credentials, the doctors could sue them, on various grounds. That would subject the governing boards to the process known as "discovery" whereby the defendants would have to disclose a wealth of documents and be subject to depositions under oath with potential perjury charges for lying. Such lawsuits have the potential to open up a big can of worms that could result in potential liability (and possible criminal prosecution as well).

If such cases were brought in the right courts, where they are more likely to have a judge who is not controlled or intimidated by the wealthy elites, the governing boards might regret ever imposing any "gag orders" and threatening punitive action against outspoken doctors who dared to violate them. What if there were class action lawsuits brought by multiple physician-plaintiffs against these governing boards? What if there were even the possibility of punitive damages, as suggested by attorney Reiner Fuellmich in another context? Would such actions diminish the governing boards' ability to intimidate all health care professionals?

This war has reached a tipping point. What is at stake is far greater than many doctors' medical licenses, credentials or their livelihoods. Never have our lives, our nation and the world been so much at risk. The boards' actions against doctors are part of the "spiritual war."

Dr. Stella Immanuel, quoted earlier in Part 1, has had much experience with "spiritual warfare." In her book *Let America Live*,[623] she describes in greater detail the spiritual issues behind "all things COVID," how she recognized them, and how God empowers His people to win the spiritual war against evil in whatever arena they are called to fight in. She also confirms how ***all*** of the damage done by COVID and the "vaccines" **can be overcome** through the power of God. Many other health care professionals share this belief. We hope that is an encouragement to everyone.

The wealthy elites have their "Great Reset," which they are desperately seeking to move forward at an accelerated pace. As of the fall of 2022, it may seem in the natural realm that those on the side of evil are winning. Everything that can be shaken is being shaken. But do not fear. God has His own "reset," but His is a "Great Awakening." It is the opposite of the elites' Great Reset. In the spiritual realm, God has already won this war. He **will** triumph over evil in the earth as well, though things will probably get worse before they get better. If you have read this far in this book, it is probably because He is awakening ***you*** in new ways, and not just to the truth about the COVID shots, but also to the truth about ***Him***, His true nature and the incredible blessings available to those who are in right standing with Him. Only through Him can we have peace without fear in the midst of the storms and chaos of life.

The same people who lied to the world about COVID have also lied about God, to keep people from knowing Him and all that He offers, which the world desperately needs right now. They have also lied about His ultimate judgment for those who are not in right standing with Him. That right standing only comes through repentance from living our lives in ways that seem right to us, but are not right with Him. He will hold each one of us accountable. His justice requires it.

But the very good news is that He makes it possible for all to easily get right with Him and have a fresh start with a "clean slate." He is calling us into a relationship with Him through Jesus to freely receive forgiveness by His amazing grace, based on the price Jesus has already paid on our behalf, so that we do not have to suffer His judgment. There is nothing anyone has done that is so bad that God will not forgive. Jesus is often referred to as "The Great Physician" as He is able to heal and cleanse our bodies of anything that ought not be there. Those who have administered, recommended, or received the shots can be totally forgiven and healed. Those who did not can also receive forgiveness for things they need to repent of and receive any needed healing as well. Then one of God's promises in the Scriptures is this:

> "If My people who are called by My name will humble themselves, and pray and seek My face, and turn from their wicked ways, then I will hear from heaven, and will forgive their sin and heal their land."[624]

*Can we, as a nation, as well as individually afford **not** to get right with God in these chaotic, unpredictable and rapidly changing times?*

---

[621] Israeli Holocaust Survivor Vera Sharav and Dr. Reiner Fuellmich Talk 'Global Genocide,' https://www.bitchute.com/video/KYbfbEfg2n98/ (March 26, 2021)

[622] https://leohohmann.files.wordpress.com/2022/01/icc-complaint-7.pdf

[623] Stella Immanuel, MD, *Let America Live* (2021)

[624] 2 Chronicles 7:14. Scripture taken from the New King James Version®. Copyright © 1982 by Thomas Nelson. Used by permission. All rights reserved.

**IF YOU WOULD LIKE TO RECEIVE
PRAYER for HEALING (for yourself or others)
or HELP in CONNECTING with GOD:**

Email Sally: info@BreakthroughsForLife.com

Subject Line: either Healing *or* Connecting (or *both*)

Chapter 46
Conclusion

We realize that the evidence presented in this book may be very difficult for many to accept or to deal with. It has been extremely challenging on the other side as well, to write about what we felt health care professionals, as well as others, needed to know. Thankfully, history teaches us that truth ultimately prevails over lies, and good triumphs over evil, just as light always overcomes the darkness.

Despite all of the difficult revelations in this book, we cannot emphasize enough that no one has to live their life overcome by fear, anxiety, depression, or other negative emotions. Help is available for every kind of problem, whether physical, emotional, mental or otherwise, even though it may not be from sources that medical professionals or their patients are used to relying on.

Since COVID began, the globalist elites' true colors have begun to show like never before. They have blinded the eyes and conditioned the minds of tens of millions of Americans, and countless others around the world, by constant lies that were too big *not* to believe, just as Hitler taught and did. **Even many of the most highly educated people have trouble believing anything contrary to the official narrative, no matter how much data or incriminating evidence is presented.**

If you have read this entire book, it should be clear that the elites' goal to inject everyone with these COVID shots is not about science or public health. It should also be clear why they demonized and refused to approve effective treatment protocols for COVID, why they have ignored all of the warning signals in the VAERS database, and why they have lied about "all things COVID."

The deception and propaganda of their official narrative that the COVID shots are "safe and effective," as well as necessary, has devastated countless millions of Americans and their families. Excess deaths are skyrocketing, The military and the workforce are being decimated. Pregnant women are losing

CONCLUSION

their babies. Infertility is increasing. Cardiovascular problems, among other diseases, are wreaking havoc among teens and young adults. Now the elites are moving quickly and relentlessly to inject children and even young babies! The genetic consequences of injecting our youth and others of reproductive age with these shots could have devastating effects on future generations – ***absent divine intervention.***

By the time you are reading this, the COVID vaccines may have already ended. However, the lessons to be learned from this chapter of history are timeless and broad in scope. Among other things, they should raise reg flags about all other "vaccines" and other drugs and products coming from Big Pharma, especially the most recent and new ones yet to come.

This book has raised many questions, including several that relate to the future of health care delivery. One thing is clear: this era of COVID has demonstrated that the current system of government-controlled health care and the current state of regulation over the pharmaceutical industry is a disaster for both providers and patients. The only ones who benefit are those in bed with the wealthy elites and those willing to support or go along with their agenda. Trust has been destroyed on several levels. In order to "stop the bleeding" from the devastating consequences of "all things COVID," it is critical to become aware of what the medical industrial complex has NOT been telling us and start questioning the official narrative on *all* major issues, not just COVID and the vaccines.

We can win this war and get on the road to recovery, both individually and collectively. Each of us has a role to play in stopping this evil agenda, even if only by refusing to go along with it. Each of us also has a role to play in helping people whose lives have been turned upside down by "all things COVID." But because this is a ***spiritual war***, we believe it cannot be won without God's intervention, mercy and grace. That will require everyone, not just health care professionals, to decide if they want to be on the side of *"playing God,"* or on the side of *connecting with God,* allowing Him to work in them and through them, and learning how to deal with the spiritual battles of life.

The quote from Dr. Lee Merritt, expressed at the beginning of Part 4, sets the stage for the choice that we all have to make:

"If you think we're fighting a virus, you're going to act like a victim.
If you think we're fighting a war, you're going to act like a warrior."

Chapter 47
Call to Action From Two Doctors on the Front Lines

"Those who will not take a stand for something will fall for anything."
Original author unknown

*Dr. Deborah Viglione and Dr. James A. Thorp are two among the countless other physicians already on the frontlines of this war. Below is their **Call to Action** to those in the health care community.*

This war is one that everyone is involved in, whether we want to be or not. No one, especially those of us in the health care community, can sit this war out on the sidelines, and there is no fence to sit on. If you choose to not get involved and not take a stand, your choice will be made for you by default. That default choice is the side of the globalist elites, and whatever the consequences of that choice are. You can no longer claim that "you did not know." This is a war *we absolutely can win,* if enough of us take a firm stand together. We are calling on you to join those of us already in the fight.

The medical community has been through a terrible ordeal already, but remember that Dr. Michael Yeadon, the former Pfizer V.P., has warned us to be "hypervigilant" about what the globalists may try to do next. They have more "pandemics" and "health emergencies" planned. ***Their agenda will only be stopped when enough people, especially in the health care community, think critically, question the official narrative on every major issue, and say "NO" to more injections, whether they are called COVID, monkeypox, or by any other name.***

The response of health care professionals plays a crucial part in determining their success. How many more people will suffer injury or die from these shots depends in large part *on us.* The elites can only succeed to the extent we allow them and help them. Now that you know the truth, the ultimate price to be paid by those who cower to the elites' fear-mongering and intimidation will be much greater than any sacrifice made in the fight against them right now.

CALL TO ACTION

They have already started on the next "emergency." If they have not been stopped by the time you are reading this, the government's new strategy of authorizing any newly formulated COVID vaccines *without any new clinical trials* will take their already harmful drug experiments to new levels of unknown dangers.

Will you be part of the solution? Will you join us and thousands of other medical professionals in questioning the official narrative on *every major issue*, and to read and think critically when presented with "medical data?"

Will you be courageous and take a stand, even if it requires sacrifice? If you are pressured to practice your profession in ways you now know are not best for your patients, and are contrary to your ethics and professional judgment, **will you speak up?** Continuing to "do what you are told," ignoring the scientific evidence, and believing the narrative without questioning it only serves to further empower and advance the elites' evil agenda. We believe that inaction or "going along" is choosing the wrong side of history.

If you think this is not affecting your life right now:

- *Do you believe that your own freedom is not worth fighting for?*
- *Are your children's and grandchildren's futures worth fighting for?*
- *Are you willing to settle for leaving a legacy as a victim who chose not to fight, or would you rather be remembered as someone who had the courage to take a stand for freedom and truth?*

As fellow health care professionals, we are calling on you to take action. Below are several ways you can make a difference within your sphere of influence:

- Will you cease to recommend or administer the current and any future reformulated COVID injections, even if pressured by your employer and threatened with losing your job?
- Will you educate your colleagues and patients as to the dangers of these injections, to provide them with truly informed consent?
- Will you join with other health care professionals in your facility and in your area to appeal to your employer(s) and local officials to stop all COVID shots immediately?
- Will you use your influence locally and politically to protect the children from these harmful and deadly shots?
- Will you warn pregnant and breastfeeding women of the dangers of these injections?

- Will you press for and insist on proper safety and efficacy testing of future drugs and vaccines and insist on transparency and release of the data?
- Will you do your duty to report possible and probable "vaccine" related adverse effects to the VAERS database?
- Will you educate yourself on effective treatment protocols for COVID-19, learn new and effective ways to treat those injured by the COVID "vaccines" and teach others the same?
- Will you educate your colleagues, patients, and others that the *unvaccinated* are not a threat and should not be criticized, demeaned or discriminated against?
- Will you speak out against "vaccine passports," any form of "digital ID under the skin" and all restrictions associated with them?
- Will you speak out against "vaccine" mandates and write medical exemptions for your patients?
- Will you appropriately record a "vaccine" injury or death in patients' medical records?
- Will you refuse to report people as "unvaccinated" if they have received at least one COVID shot?
- Will you speak out against mandatory masking and masking in schools?
- Will you speak out against asymptomatic testing?

Public officials and others:
- Will you establish procedures to protect local blood supplies from COVID-vaccinated blood?
- Will you work with health care professionals in your area to establish a vaccine injury hot line?
- Will you investigate 5G and the health consequences of its use and take appropriate action?
- Will you encourage people to report to you and law enforcement if they are being pressured or coerced to get the COVID shots or threatened with consequences for refusing them?

WHICH SIDE OF HISTORY DO YOU WANT TO BE ON?

Which will you choose to be: a victim or a warrior?

"You may choose to look the other way, but you can never say again that you did not know."

William Wilberforce

ABOUT THE AUTHORS

SALLY SAXON, J.D., is a graduate of Northwestern University School of Law in Chicago. She is a retired attorney who worked for one of the biggest law firms in Seattle for several years. She also had her own practice for three years before leaving her law career to pursue other interests. For approximately two years, she also served as the Executive Director of the Northwest Legal Foundation, an organization devoted to fighting unlawful and abusive government actions. Sally also lived in China for four years, teaching English and studying Chinese. She comes from a family of health care professionals, which was a key factor in deciding to write this book. She is also the author of *Globalists on Trial: The Hidden Agenda to Destroy America From Within* (originally published in 2020, under a different subtitle, with an Updated & Expanded version to be released in mid-2023). She has also taught classes on various subjects related to empowering women over 50, and challenging others to do things they never thought they could. Sally is also a minister with the Christian International network, is actively involved in ministry and has seen the miracle-working power of God transform many lives.

DEBORAH VIGLIONE, MD is a board-certified internist who has practiced medicine since 1986. She received a Military Professional Scholarship and her medical degree from the University of North Carolina at Chapel Hill. She completed her Internal Medicine Residency with the U. S. Air Force at Keesler AFB, MS and was on active duty in the Air Force for a little over 11 years. She is an active freedom fighter in Northwest Florida, organized the Panhandle Doctors for Truth, and has held freedom rallies with thousands in attendance, as well as a freedom doctor educational conference. Dr. Viglione is a leader in the field of nutrigenomics and methylation She received her Board Certification in Anti-Aging Medicine from the American Academy of Anti-Aging and Regenerative Medicine in 2012 along with a Stem Cell Fellowship. She has been practicing Integrative and Anti-Aging Medicine since 1994 and maintains a very busy practice in that field at Living Waters Regenerative Medicine Center in Gulf Breeze, Florida.

JAMES A. THORP, MD is a Board-Certified Obstetrician Gynecologist and Maternal Fetal Medicine Physician with over 43 years of obstetrical experience. While serving as a very busy clinician his entire career he has also been very active in clinical research with about 200 publications. He has seen over 22,800 high risk pregnancies in the past three years. He has served as a reviewer for major medical journals, has served on the Board of Directors for the Society of Maternal Fetal Medicine, and also served the American Board of Obstetrics & Gynecology. He served in the United States Air Force as an Obstetrician Gynecologist, having been awarded a Health Professions Scholarship for his medical school education. Dr. Thorp testified in the US Senate under the Bush administration in 2003 for his expertise in treating the fetus as a patient with in-utero therapies. Most recently Dr. Thorp has focused his research efforts on the COVID-19 pandemic and published several peer-reviewed scientific publications documenting the dangers of the vaccine in women of reproductive age and in pregnancy. His publications conclusively demonstrate that the COVID-19 "vaccination" experiment has been one of the greatest disasters in the history of medicine. Dr Thorp has clearly shown the mass death from COVID-19 pandemic that would have been prevented had the healthcare system and governmental agencies NOT prevented the widespread support of early and safe treatments proven successful by multiple experts around the world.

Contact the authors

Through the website: www.SallySaxon.com

or

Sally Saxon, JD: info@BreakthroughsForLife.com

Deborah Viglione, MD: debviglione@gmail.com

James A. Thorp, MD: jathorpMFM@gmail.com

Thank you for reading our book!
May we ask a simple favor?

If you found value in this book, would you kindly write **VERY SHORT 1 or 2 SENTENC** **BOOK REVIEW ON AMAZON or** **at least leave a star-rating?**

You can even leave a review under a "nickname" if you want to.

Thanks so much for helping to spread the word.

For more info on the

Updated & Expanded Edition *of Sally's book,*

GLOBALISTS on TRIAL
The Hidden Agenda to Destroy America From Within

expected to be published in mid-2023, go to:

www.GlobalistsOnT

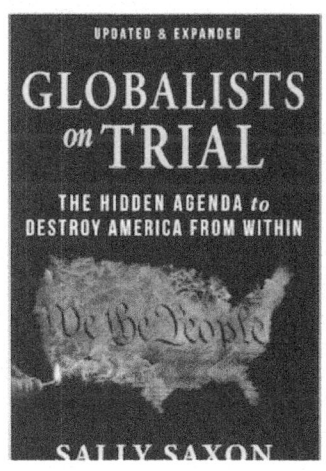

Made in the USA
Las Vegas, NV
11 May 2023

71866463R00164